MOLECULES AND MENTAL ILLNESS

Samuel H. Barondes

**SCIENTIFIC
AMERICAN
LIBRARY**

A division of HPHLP
New York

Library of Congress Cataloging-in-Publication Data
Barondes, Samuel H., 1933–
    Molecules and mental illness / Samuel H. Barondes.
       p.   cm.
    Includes bibliographical references and index.
    ISBN 0-7167-5041-4
    1. Biological psychiatry.   I. Title.
    RC341.B33   1993
    616.89—dc20   92-35150
                                                                     CIP

ISSN 1040-3213

Printed in the United States of America

Scientific American Library
A division of HPHLP
New York

Distributed by W. H. Freeman and Company.
41 Madison Avenue, New York, NY 10010
20 Beaumont Street, Oxford OXI 2NQ, England

2 3 4 5 6 7 8 9 0   KP   9 9 8 7 6 5 4 3

This book is number 44 of a series.

CONTENTS

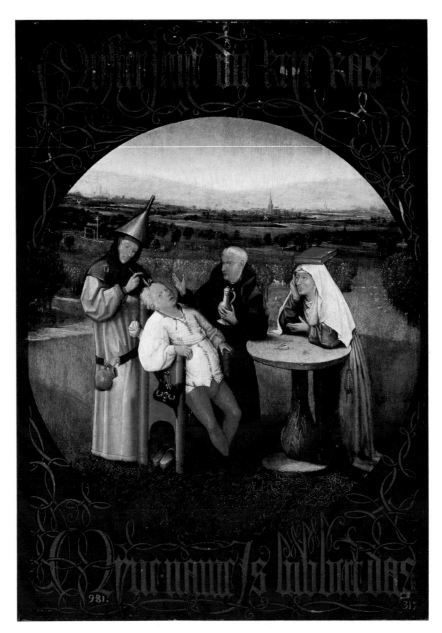

Extraction of the Stone of Folly, 1475–1480, by Hieronymus Bosch.

PREFACE

In the past few decades we have learned a great deal about proteins and nucleic acids, the molecular building blocks of all biological systems. This knowledge is being applied in many branches of medicine. The goal of this book is to show its impact on our view of mental illness and its treatment.

Until recently, few people have been thinking about the connections between molecules and mental illness, because to do this requires familiarity with two very different intellectual and professional traditions. My opportunity to combine them came during my postdoctoral training at the National Institutes of Health (NIH) between 1960 and 1963. When I arrived at NIH, I had completed medical school and was thinking of embarking on a career in psychiatry. But I also wanted to learn more about fundamental biology by working in a laboratory. At NIH I met Gordon Tomkins, who was deeply committed to relating basic science to medicine and had founded a department to achieve this goal. Gordon was bursting with knowledge and enthusiasm about the infant field of molecular biology and was convinced that it would ultimately explain almost everything (which, to me, meant even psychiatry).

To provide a taste of molecular biology, Gordon arranged for me to become the second postdoctoral fellow in the then tiny laboratory of Marshall Nirenberg. I began there immediately before Marshall's discovery that a synthetic nucleic acid, called poly U, could act as an artificial genetic message. Within months I became an industrious student of poly U, while Marshall went on to work with other synthetic nucleic acids, ultimately deciphering the genetic code by which nucleic acid sequences are translated into the language of proteins. It was obvious to me, and to everyone else, that Marshall's work was monumental; and within a few years it was honored with a Nobel prize. The experience was an extraordinarily exciting introduction to the laboratory, and supported Gordon's belief that, if you study things at the molecular level, anything is possible. I was hooked.

After a year in Gordon's laboratory in which I began to use molecular techniques to study the mechanism for storing memories in the brain, I went on to psychiatric training and have worked in both psychiatry and basic biological sciences ever since. Although the integration of these fields has progressed more slowly than I would have liked, the pace is picking up. This book is designed to provide enough essential information about biology and psychiatry for readers unfamiliar with both fields to appreciate how they are coming together.

In writing this book I have been greatly aided by the advice of many colleagues and friends and have enjoyed the benefit of working with an extraordinary group of professionals at Scientific American Library. Two people I wish to single out for special thanks are my editor, Sonia DiVittorio, and my assistant Anne Poirier, who each made invaluable contributions. My daughters Elizabeth and Jessica, both more comfortable with words than with molecules, were often my target audience. "Recapitulation (in Verse)" is especially for them. I hope you like it too.

Samuel H. Barondes
Sausalito, California
October 1992

For
Elizabeth Francesca
and
Jessica Gabrielle

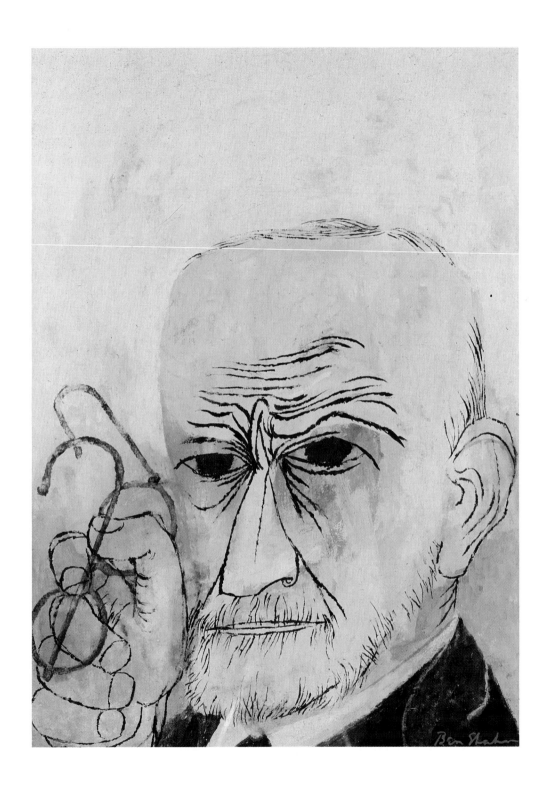

THE EVOLUTION OF
BIOLOGICAL PSYCHIATRY

Psychiatry is the branch of medicine concerned with disorders of human behavior. Some of these result primarily from psychological experiences, others from biological factors. Whereas all psychiatrists recognize both etiologies, many concentrate on a particular one. Those who are more interested in biological causes and pharmacological treatments than in psychological and social ones define their perspective as neuropsychiatry or, as here, biological psychiatry.

It will surprise many readers to learn that some psychiatrists have such a frankly biological point of view. This is because most psychiatrists they know about tend to work with psychological tools, in the service of patients whose primary goal is to master their individual limitations or their difficulties in interpersonal relationships. But psychiatry also grapples with

--------- OPPOSITE: Portrait of Sigmund Freud by Ben Shahn. ---------

a set of far graver problems whose analysis and treatment depend, in part, on a biological approach. These include profound disturbances in mood such as manic-depressive illness and major depression; disabling conditions characterized by high levels of anxiety such as panic disorder, agoraphobia, and obsessive-compulsive disorder; and a particularly devastating mental illness called schizophrenia.

These disorders are of great interest to psychiatrists not only because of their seriousness, but also because they are remarkably common. At least one in ten people will be directly affected by one of them. It is actually rare to find anyone whose close family or friends are untouched.

Of course the growing role of biology in understanding and treating these disorders in no way negates the importance of psychological and social factors. In psychiatric illnesses, as with other human infirmities, a combination of biological and behavioral factors may contribute to the development of symptoms. For example, consider diabetes, a complex metabolic disorder in which a critical feature is inefficient glucose utilization. In certain forms of diabetes abnormal genes lead to impaired functioning of the hormone insulin, which is needed to metabolize glucose properly. The genetic predisposition is necessary for development of this type of diabetes. But it is not sufficient. In order to display altered sugar metabolism, such patients must usually be somewhat obese. Their obesity, in turn, tends to result from a combination of psychological and cultural factors. For this reason treatment may combine medications that directly influence glucose metabolism with psychological techniques that facilitate weight control. In many instances the latter are sufficient to ameliorate this genetically based physical illness.

In trying to solve complicated medical problems, be they diabetes or schizophrenia, it is most practical to concentrate on those variables that lend themselves best to scientific investigation and that point to effective treatments. In the case of American psychiatry, perceptions of the practicality of the different approaches have been in flux. Early in this century, when biology seemed too arcane, psychological factors were emphasized. However, in the past few decades the biological approach to psychiatry has attracted increasing support.

There are several reasons for the current popularity of the biological approach. On the negative side is an intense frustration with the limited success of psychological treatments for serious mental disorders, such as schizophrenia, a frustration expressed most forcefully by disappointed parents of young patients afflicted with these conditions. They feel especially aggrieved at psychological theorists for unjustifiably holding them responsible for their children's maladies. On the positive side, hopes have been raised by advances in biological psychiatry, such as the considerable progress in developing successful pharmacological treatments for an increasing number of disorders. Furthermore, the recent burst of knowledge in the fields of genetics, molecular biology, and neuroscience has begun to yield important insights that are applicable to psychiatry. It now seems reasonable to expect that a more powerful biology will provide the tools to solve some of psychiatry's most refractory problems.

The purpose of this chapter is to recount several critical events in the early history of biological psychiatry that illustrate both its limitations and its practical value. To put this in perspective, I will begin by describing the struggle of the young Sigmund Freud, late in the nineteenth century, to choose between a biological and a psychological approach to psychiatry. I will then review some important biomedical discoveries made in the first half of the twentieth century that led to the eradication of two important psychiatric disorders of that time.

Freud Abandons Biological Psychiatry

To put present developments in their historical context it is important to recognize that this is not the first time that a biological approach has played a dominant role in psychiatry. A similar interest was sparked in the middle of the nineteenth century by the development of techniques to study normal and pathological brain anatomy. Even with the limitations of the gross tools of brain dissection and light microscopy available then, much was learned about brain structure and the localization of behavioral functions, such as vision and movement, to particular neuronal circuits in the brain.

These exciting discoveries inspired a young medical student, Sigmund Freud (1856–1939), who was enrolled at the University of Vienna, where much of this work was being done. At the age of 20, Freud began research on the microscopic structure of nerve cells, while working in the laboratory of Ernst Brücke (1819–1892), a leading neuroscientist of the period. Along with the German physicist Hermann von Helmholtz, Brücke pioneered the idea that the principles of the physical sciences could be applied to an understanding of the function of the brain.

Drawing done by Freud in 1878 of neurons in spinal ganglia of a fish.

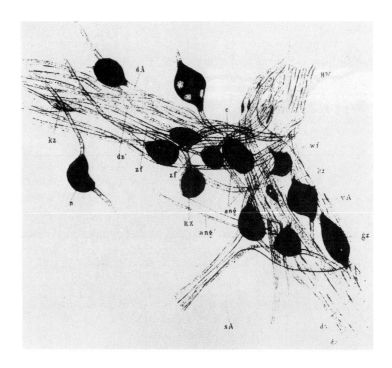

Under Brücke's tutelage Freud made fundamental studies of the development and cellular organization of the nervous system in fish. While completing his clinical training, Freud extended his studies to the human brain. This work was done in the Laboratory of Cerebral Anatomy in Vienna under the direction of Theodor Meynert, a prominent neuroanatomist and psychiatrist. Freud also undertook innovative psychopharmacological studies, investigating the behavioral effects of cocaine.

It was Freud's hope to use such approaches to understand normal and pathological behavior in terms of biological mechanisms, goals he maintained for two decades, and explicitly expressed at the age of 39 in his *Project for a Scientific Psychology* (1895) which begins as follows:

> The intention is to furnish a psychology that shall be a natural science: that is, to represent psychical processes as quantitatively determinate states of specifiable material particles, thus making those processes perspicuous and free from contradiction.

Freud had in mind that the units of this natural science, the "specifiable material particles," would be neurons, the cells of the nervous system, whose structure and organization he helped to elucidate while working with Brücke. He recognized that the transmission of signals between neurons was the basis of behavior, and that changes in the strength of neuronal connections might underlie the adaptive process that constitutes learning and memory. But, after devoting many years to this approach, Freud reluctantly came to believe that the available tools were not adequate for the task.

For some years he had also been interested in psychology, beginning in 1885 when he came under the influence of Jean-Martin Charcot (1825–1893), a leading Parisian neurologist. Charcot, at that time, was especially concerned with patients, virtually all young women, who presented patterns of muscle paralysis that did not appear to be due to damaged nerves or muscles. Another distinguishing symptom, designated "la belle indifference," was their remarkable lack of concern with their disability. The overall picture suggested that this was primarily a psychological problem, and at the time was called hysteria. Today it is called conversion disorder,

Jean-Martin Charcot discussing a patient with hysteria.

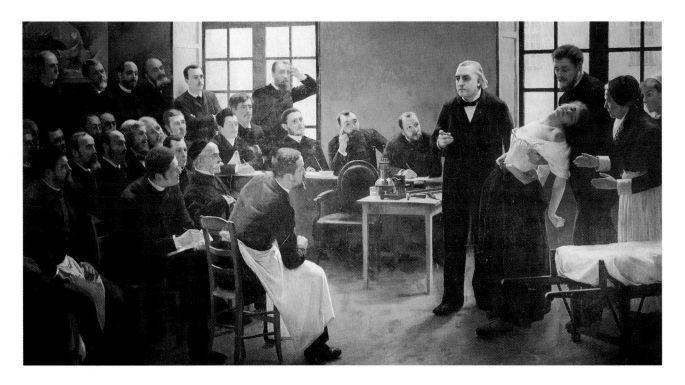

A late-nineteenth-century demonstration of the medical use of hypnosis.

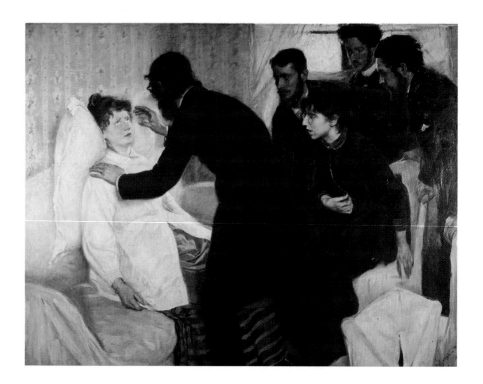

because the patient presumably "converts" psychological conflicts into physical symptoms. The paralysis was of especial interest to Charcot since he found that this particular symptom could be dramatically alleviated by a psychological technique, hypnosis. To a neurologist accustomed to dealing with incurable physical maladies frequently due to irreversible degenerative processes, the lure of a reversible disorder that responded to a simple treatment was hard to resist.

For Freud the study of hysterical paralysis was additionally attractive because it allowed him to work at the intersection between the physical and mental realms, albeit in a different way than he had originally envisioned. Initially he had been interested in behaviors controlled by biological processes. In ancient times physicians had actually concocted a biological explanation for hysteria, attributing it to the wandering of the uterus, which gave the syndrome its name (from the Greek *hystera*, for womb). What Freud recognized was the difficulty of replacing such nonsense with biological insights that could be taken more seriously. In fact his work with hysteria led him away from an interest in how the brain begets

Chapter 1

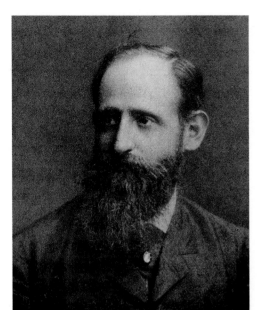

Josef Breuer.

the mind to how the mind controls the body. He was particularly attracted to this alternative question because he could pursue it in the context of his clinical practice, obviating the need for both a university position and laboratory facilities that were very scarce. Clinical practice had the added advantage that it made it easier to support his wife and six children, the first born when Freud was 31.

The evolution of Freud's work on hysteria was very much influenced by a senior colleague in Vienna, Josef Breuer (1842–1925). Like Freud, Breuer began his career with an interest in neuroscience but then moved to clinical practice. Among his patients was Bertha Pappenheim, whose identity was, during her lifetime, disguised by the pseudonym "Anna O." She was a twenty-one-year-old woman who suffered from paralysis and diminished sensation in an arm and leg and had lost the ability to speak her native German. Conducting conversations with her in English, which she continued to speak fluently, Breuer found that her symptoms would vanish as Anna talked about past events that led up to them. It was this procedure, which Anna called (in English) the "talking cure," that seemed to be

Bertha Pappenheim, the patient Breuer referred to as "Anna O."

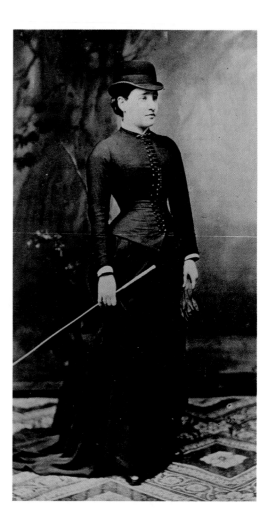

therapeutically effective, rather than the hypnosis, which Breuer also used. After two years of daily meetings the patient's paralysis subsided and her ability to speak German returned. This dramatic recovery was attributed to Breuer's improvised therapeutic technique, which was the forerunner of psychoanalysis.

After experimenting with variants of Breuer's method to treat several other young women with similar symptoms, Freud accepted his new calling. What he had found was an illness that could be ameliorated with a psychological approach. Determining how that treatment worked and the psychological basis of the hysterical disorder replaced the less clinically relevant cellular neuroscience that had captivated him for many years.

Freud's change of attitude is documented in *Studies on Hysteria*, which, like *Project for a Scientific Psychology*, was written in 1895:

> I have not always been a psychotherapist. Like other neuro-pathologists, I was trained to employ local diagnoses and electro-prognosis* and it still strikes me myself as strange that the case histories I write should read like short stories and that, as one might say, they lack the serious stamp of science. I must console myself with the reflection that the nature of the subject is evidently responsible for this, rather than any preference of my own. The fact is that local diagnosis and electrical reactions lead nowhere in the study of hysteria, whereas a detailed description of mental processes such as we are accustomed to find in the works of imaginative writers enables me, with the use of a few psychological formulas, to obtain at least some kind of insight into the course of that affection.

In responding to the puzzle of hysterical paralysis, Freud had given up biological psychiatry and begun to invent psychoanalysis.

The Serious Stamp of Science

If one accepts that a person can become paralyzed or lose the ability to converse in his or her native tongue for psychological reasons, one next must ask, how can this come about? For Breuer the task of answering this question seemed too great. But to Freud it was a challenge worth taking. And, as quoted above, he was comfortable using "a few psychological formulas" so that he might obtain "at least some kind of insight" even though the work might "lack the serious stamp of science."

What Freud inferred from intensive examination of his patients' thoughts and dreams was that hysterical paralysis was related to unexpressed sexual impulses. Since the patients did not directly reveal this connection, he concluded that the impulses had been repressed and relegated from the conscious to the unconscious cognitive domain. Repression was presumably necessary as a self-protective defense against the pain that acknowledging these impulses would cause. But why were such natural impulses painful?

---

*Terms presumably meaning cellular and electrophysiological analysis.

Chronology of Freud's Early Career

1856 Born May 6.

1873 Entered University of Vienna as a medical student.

1876 Began working on the structure of nerve cells at Ernst Brücke's Institute of Physiology.

1878 Published significant discoveries on the anatomy of the nervous system of a fish.

1881 Became a demonstrator at Brücke's Institute.

1883 Worked at the Psychiatric Clinic of the General Hospital in Vienna and the Laboratory of Cerebral Anatomy with Theodor Meynert.

1884 Investigated uses of cocaine both as a local anesthetic and stimulant, to his later regret resisting evidence that cocaine was addictive.

1885 Went to Paris to study with Jean-Martin Charcot; became interested in hysteria.

1886 Began private practice, specializing in diseases of the nervous system.

1887 Experimented with hypnosis.

1891 Published his first book, *Aphasia*, a neurological work.

1895 Wrote *Project for a Scientific Psychology*, which was not published until after his death. Published *Studies in Hysteria* with Josef Breuer, which laid the foundation of psychoanalysis.

Freud speculated that the emotional pain arose because normal sexual impulses had been linked in the mind with traumatic events in childhood. But what was the nature of the trauma? Initially Freud suspected actual sexual abuse. Lacking clear evidence he then settled on fantasized sexual abuse and premature sexual stimulation. The battle between the pent up sexual forces that resulted and the repressive defenses erected to restrain them were, in this view, the cause of the hysterical symptoms. Successful treatment resolved this battle by providing insight within the context of the special relationship between analyst and analysand. The pent up forces were released. The symptoms subsided. The patient was cured.

This simplified summary attempts to capture Freud's approach to this challenging problem, but it is difficult to be accurate since his ideas kept changing rapidly during his early studies of hysteria, and continued to change throughout his lifetime. In retrospect, one of Freud's biggest mistakes was to underemphasize the importance of a sustained pattern of actual, rather than fantasized, childhood sexual abuse and trauma, which we now know to play an important role in the genesis of many behavioral abnormalities. In spite of this and other limitations, the fact remains that Freud, empowered by some clinical success and gifted with a rich imagination and a captivating literary style, could elaborate his insights and speculations so persuasively that they came to dominate psychiatry.

Although these simple early speculations launched Freud on a career of extraordinary influence, he never really forgot the limitations of his new approach. Time and again he reminded his readers of his own awareness that his work lacked "the serious stamp of science," which awaited advances in biology that had not yet been achieved. For example, in *Beyond the Pleasure Principle*, published in 1920, he insists that "the deficiencies in our description would probably vanish if we were already in a position to replace the psychological terms by physiological or chemical ones." Twenty-five years after *Project for a Scientific Psychology*, he still looked forward to a psychiatry that would actually explain psychological processes through biological mechanisms.

Curing Mental Symptoms by Curing Brain Diseases

While Freud was developing psychoanalysis, biomedical scientists were making great progress in understanding and treating several major psychiatric disorders. But the biological approach that they used was quite different from the one that Freud had envisioned. He wanted to know how the brain functioned to generate behavior, which would presumably lead to a general understanding of psychopathology. They tackled psychiatric syn-

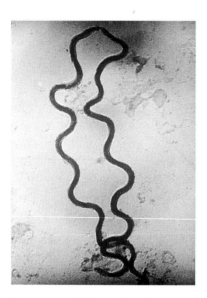

Treponema pallidum, the microorganism that causes syphilis.

dromes that turned out to be major manifestations of recognized physical diseases. If the physical disease were cured, the behavioral abnormalities would vanish.

Most dramatic among their successes was the discovery of the cause of a very prevalent mental illness of the day, called general paresis, or general paralysis of the insane, which afflicted about 10 percent to 15 percent of patients in psychiatric hospitals at the turn of the century. It is a progressive disease that often begins with symptoms of mania, a pattern of behavior that includes excitement, euphoria, and grandiose delusions. Within months to years patients then typically go on to develop the cognitive deterioration and the paralysis that together were its hallmark. During the last half of the nineteenth century many leading psychiatrists considered the disorder to be due to psychological factors. In fact, learned debates about the etiology of general paresis were a major preoccupation of psychiatrists during this period.

A triumph of the biology of the early twentieth century was the demonstration that general paresis was in fact a late manifestation of syphilis, a venereal disease caused by infection with the spirochete *Treponema pallidum.* This microorganism persists in the human body for many years and ultimately invades the nervous system. Manic behavior and dementia may not develop until many years after the initial infection. This long lag between infection by *T. pallidum* and development of behavioral symptoms was, in fact, the major obstacle to relating them. One famous victim, Lord Randolph Churchill, father of Winston Churchill, did not succumb for more than two decades after contracting the venereal disease.

To appreciate the importance of syphilis a century ago, one might view it as the AIDS of that time. Both are fatal infectious diseases caused by microorganisms that can be transmitted sexually. Both are chronic diseases with long incubation periods when the patient is free of symptoms. Both ultimately infect the nervous system, often to produce progressive dementia.

General paresis provides a model not only of diagnostic success but also of rational development of a cure. For once *T. pallidum* was discovered early in this century, attention could be diverted from looking for psychological remedies to seeking the means of eradicating the causative agent. This goal led the German microbiologist Paul Ehrlich (1854–1915), a major figure in the creation of modern pharmacology, to establish a systematic approach to development of therapeutic drugs.

The first step necessary was to find an experimental animal that could be infected with *T. pallidum,* so that treatments could be tested. This posed a transient stumbling block since, like many microorganisms, *T. pallidum* is

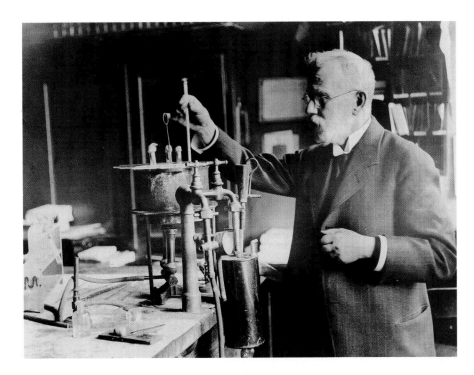

The momentous discovery of a pharmacological treatment for syphilis was celebrated in the 1940 motion picture *Dr. Ehrlich's Magic Bullet*. Paul Ehrlich *(top)* was portrayed by Edward G. Robinson *(bottom)*.

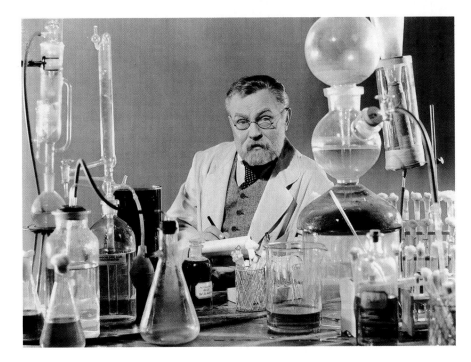

The Evolution of Biological Psychiatry

Discovering the Nature, Cause, and Cure
of General Paresis

1672   Thomas Willis, an English physician and neuroanatomist, called attention to a class of patients who developed symptoms of "stupidity and foolishness" and "would afterwards fall into paralysis which [Willis] was even in the habit of predicting."

Late 1700s   Reports appeared emphasizing the correlation between paralysis, insanity, and mania.

Mid 1800s   Many reports appeared that patients with general paresis had previously been infected with syphilis, suggesting that it might be the cause.

1867   Wilhelm Griesinger, a very influential German psychiatrist and physiologist, resisted the increasing suggestions that syphilis was the cause of general paresis, although he noted that affected men were frequently sexually promiscuous.

1904   Alois Alzheimer, the German neuropathologist (who also discovered the dementing illness that bears his name), presented a full description of the microscopic changes in the brains of patients with general paresis.

1906   August von Wassermann, a German microbiologist, developed a blood test for syphilis, which established that patients with general paresis were infected with the veneral disease.

1910   Paul Ehrlich, a German microbiologist and Nobel laureate (1908, for earlier work on immunology), developed arsphenamine, the "magic bullet," to kill the causative microorganism.

1913   Hideyo Noguchi, a Japanese microbiologist, directly demonstrated the microorganism *T. pallidum* in the brain of patients with neurosyphilis and developed methods for its cultivation in test tubes.

1917   Julius Wagner-Jauregg, a Viennese psychiatrist, produced lasting remissions of general paresis by deliberately infecting patients with malaria, inducing fevers that killed the microorganism (Nobel prize, 1927).

1928   Alexander Fleming, a British microbiologist, discovered the antibacterial action of penicillin (Nobel prize, 1945).

1943   Penicillin was increasingly used for infectious diseases and ultimately virtually eradicated neurosyphilis.

$$HCl \cdot H_2N \quad\quad\quad\quad\quad NH_2 \cdot HCl$$

$$HO-\!\!\!\!\bigcirc\!\!\!\!-As\!=\!As-\!\!\!\!\bigcirc\!\!\!\!-OH$$

Arsphenamine

somewhat selective for its normal host. Eventually, however, infections were established in rabbits. Then the search began for a drug that would eradicate the infection without damaging the rabbits.

After a long series of unsuccessful tests, Ehrlich finally discovered a compound that met both criteria, one of the hundreds of arsenic-containing chemicals that he examined. The drug was arsphenamine (better known as Salvarsan). It became famous as Dr. Ehrlich's "magic bullet," so called because it found its way to the invading microorganism and destroyed it without damaging the tissues of the host. Furthermore, arsphenamine proved effective not only in rabbits but also in patients with syphilis. A specific and effective treatment had been devised.

Unfortunately, the "magic" worked only in early stages of syphilitic infection. By killing *T. pallidum* in the blood, arsphenamine could prevent the brain from being infected, so new cases of general paresis became less common. But if a brain infection was already established, the drug could not eradicate it because it could not adequately penetrate into the infected tissue.

The brain infection turned out to be controllable, but in an unexpected way. This was achieved by Julius Wagner-Jauregg (1857–1940), a Viennese psychiatrist (and outspoken antagonist of Freud's) who observed that patients with general paresis sometimes showed lasting improvement if they contracted an infectious disease that produced high fever. For this reason he deliberately infected patients with malaria, a disease that induces repetitive febrile episodes every few days. Although the reason for the therapeutic effect was unclear, we now know that the high body temperature is lethal for *T. pallidum* but not for the patient. This crude and inelegant treatment of one disease with another proved so important that in 1927 Wagner-Jauregg became the first psychiatrist to win a Nobel prize.

More definitive help for patients with neurosyphilis came from another unexpected source, the chance discovery by British microbiologist Alexander Fleming (1881–1955) of the antibacterial action of a chemical made by a mold. This antibiotic, penicillin, proved so efficient in killing *T. pallidum,* and so harmless to patients, that it was possible to administer doses sufficient to eradicate established brain infections. When penicillin became widely available after World War II, one of the commonest psychiatric disorders of the past century was virtually eliminated.

General paresis was not the only mental illness that was cured during this early phase of scientific medicine. Another common cause of psychiatric hospitalization early in the twentieth century, especially in the American South, was pellagra, a disorder whose behavioral manifestations included impaired reasoning, agitation, and depression. These troubling psychiatric symptoms were characteristically accompanied by physical abnormalities affecting the skin and the gastrointestinal tract.

Early in this century Joseph Goldberger (1874–1929), working in the U.S. Public Health Service, established that pellagra was due to an extreme nutritional deficiency. We now know that the missing nutrient is niacin, a B vitamin that plays a critical role in the metabolic processes of all tissues,

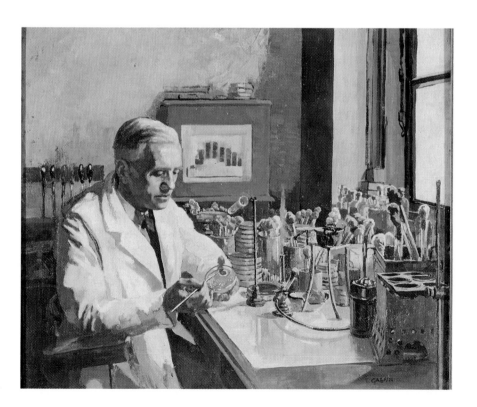

Alexander Fleming.

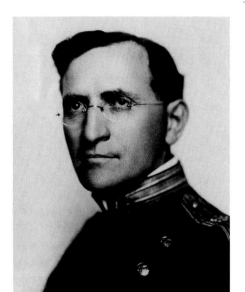

Joseph Goldberger.

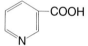

Nicotinic acid
(niacin)

including the brain. Niacin was first identified as an essential nutrient in systematic animal studies. Then human studies showed that nutritional supplements rich in niacin eliminated the symptoms of pellagra. This disease is now virtually unknown in developed societies thanks to improvements in general nutrition, including the addition of niacin to the "enriched flour" commonly used in commercial bread. This preventative measure has proven so effective that today Goldberger's great achievement in psychiatry is virtually forgotten.

The stories of general paresis and pellagra represent great successes. But there remained many other major psychiatric syndromes that seemed refractory to a biological approach. What made these disorders so difficult to investigate was that, in contrast to general paresis or pellagra, they were not accompanied by obvious biological abnormalities. In their absence, explanations and remedies based on psychological and social causes seemed plausible. Furthermore, those approaches lent themselves better to theories about behavior. In contrast, the success of biologists in preventing or treating general paresis and pellagra had not revealed a thing about the way the mind works. All that had really been established was that, for the mind to function normally, it was necessary to keep the brain well nourished with niacin and free of infection by *T. pallidum.*

The Challenge
to Biological Psychiatry

The reason that the most important psychiatric disorders of our time—major depression, schizophrenia, manic-depressive illness, and anxiety disorders—have resisted the classical biomedical approach is that they do not appear to be due to such simple exogenous factors as infection or malnutrition. As we have seen, disorders of that type lend themselves to identification of a well-defined single cause and invention of a cure. Once *T. pallidum* was discovered, ways were found to kill it. Once niacin deficiency was discovered it proved easy to remedy. In contrast, the psychiatric disorders that we will be concerned with in this book may have complex, interacting causes. These may include not only innate biological factors, but also a range of environmental ones, including culture, family structure, and physical circumstances. Their interplay shapes the brains and behavioral repertoires of all people, including psychiatric patients, as they develop through the course of their lives. Even if we were to find a single major predisposing biological factor for such conditions, it would be very difficult to undo the whole process with a single "magic bullet."

Given this complexity, it should not be surprising that much of the success in applying biological techniques to such problems has so far been at the level of developing palliative treatments rather than at the level of identifying cause and definitive cure. A great deal of progress has in fact been made in finding drugs to alleviate symptoms, beginning with a series of exciting, serendipitous discoveries, mainly in the 1950s, that suddenly provided effective drugs for depression, anxiety, mania, and psychotic behavior. The results, in turn, stimulated intense interest in the mechanism of action of these drugs in the brain.

These drugs provided a number of avenues of further progress. First, they facilitated discovery of many important brain chemicals, with which they interact, that play important roles in brain signaling. Identification of these chemicals, called neurotransmitters and receptors, has, in turn, provided the basis for more rational drug design, which is gradually leading to the development of better symptomatic treatments. Finally, analysis of the effects of these drugs on the neurotransmitters and receptors has provided some clues to innate abnormalities in brain chemistry that may underlie or predispose to certain symptoms of mental illness.

But the promise of even greater progress has come from another source: the remarkable advances in genetics in the past few decades. The enormous power of this ongoing work now makes it possible for the first time to utilize the long-established observation that psychiatric disorders run in families. Until recently genetic studies of mental illness were confined to descriptions of patterns of inheritance, because there were no established techniques to allow a search for the relevant genes. But now an effective and rapidly evolving technology makes it possible to achieve this goal. Identification of the specific genes involved in mental illness and their role in brain function will have immense theoretical and practical consequences.

The purpose of this book is to show how advances in modern biology are being applied to psychiatry. To do this it is necessary to review the status of several fields, including human genetics, molecular genetics, cellular neuroscience, and psychopharmacology, which are concerned with such questions as the ways that genes work to control nervous system function and the ways that drugs work to modulate it. The next four chapters will be devoted to this background information. The following three will then consider their application to the major problems faced by contemporary psychiatry.

In reading this book it is important to appreciate that, despite considerable progress, the problem of fully explaining behavior in biological terms, which so inspired the young Freud, remains unsolved. What has been achieved so far are powerful insights into the nature and control of the molecules and cells that are responsible for brain functions, but only a rudimentary understanding of the way these components work together to make a single mind. This is far less than Freud had desired; but far more than he ever imagined.

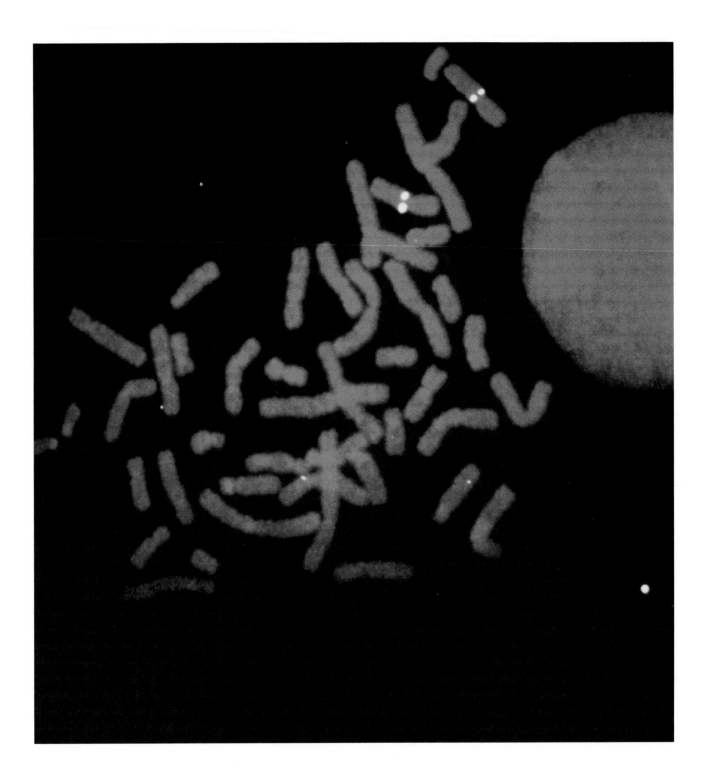

2

THE GENETICS OF BEHAVIOR

One of the principal goals of this book is to show that genes, the fundamental units of heredity, are major determinants of human conduct. In fact, there is considerable evidence that genes have a very wide sphere of behavioral influence, ranging from variations in temperament to susceptibility to certain forms of mental illness. In this chapter I will describe some basic principles that are essential for understanding how genes influence behavior.

The idea that behavioral traits can be inherited is not a new one. It was already apparent to Charles Darwin (1809–1882), as he formulated his theory of evolution. Furthermore, in *The Descent of Man and Selection in Relation to Sex* (1871), Darwin stated explicitly that behavioral tendencies were in-

OPPOSITE: Chromosomes in a human cell. Yellow dots show the location of a particular gene that is specifically expressed in muscle.

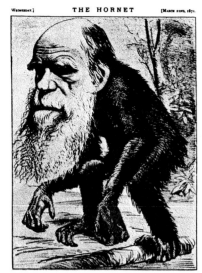

A caricature of Charles Darwin, whose view of the relationship of human to animal behavior aroused even more criticism in 1871 than it does in some quarters today.

herited not only by animals but also by people:

> So in regard to mental qualities, their transmission is manifest in our dogs, horses, and other domestic animals. Besides special tastes and habits, general intelligence, courage, bad and good temper, etc., are certainly transmitted. With man we see similar facts . . . that genius, which implies a wonderfully complex combination of high faculties, tends to be inherited; and . . . that insanity and deteriorated mental powers likewise run in families.

Although Darwin was convinced that the inheritance of behavioral tendencies was an important factor in evolution, he had no idea how the process worked. The purpose of this chapter is to describe this process by introducing the basic principles of genetics. To illustrate these principles, I will first consider several inherited human disorders that have profound mental (as well as physical) manifestations; these disorders are relatively simple examples since they are caused by an abnormality in one or both copies of a single gene. I will then proceed to studies of the inheritance of complex behavioral traits controlled either by one gene or by many acting together. These examples will show that genes can control such distinctive traits as courtship behavior and emotionality in animals, as well as components of human personality.

Huntington's Disease: Dominant Inheritance

Huntington's disease is a degenerative brain disorder that affects about 1 in 20,000 people. It results from the inheritance of a single abnormal gene and produces symptoms that include depression, personality change, impaired memory, and abnormal involuntary movements. The underlying pathology consists of the degeneration and death of nerve cells in regions of the brain concerned with control of movement and thought processes.

An important feature of Huntington's disease is that it does not strike until middle age, which illustrates the critical point that a particular gene, which is transmitted at conception, may exert no detectable influence for many years. It also illustrates the distinction between two important concepts in genetics: genotype and phenotype. Genotype is the genetic composition of the individual, whereas phenotype is the observable expression of a particular gene or genes. People born with the defective gene responsible for Huntington's disease have a genotype that includes this property from the moment of conception; but they do not have the phenotype of Huntington's disease until they begin to express behavioral abnormalities.

The single abnormal (or mutant) gene that causes Huntington's disease is transmitted to offspring in a characteristic pattern. The expression of the disorder in these relatives is charted in a branching diagram called a pedigree by means of standard symbols, some of which are displayed in the figure at right. As shown in the pedigree below, this pattern, called autosomal dominant inheritance, is characterized by expression of the disease in one of the parents of an affected individual and in about half of his or her siblings and descendants.

The groundwork for understanding this and other patterns of inheritance was laid by the experiments conducted by the Austrian monk Gregor Mendel (1822–1884) in the 1860s. Mendel, by crossbreeding different strains of garden peas and observing properties such as the color and texture of their seeds, was able to infer certain formal rules of heredity. These rules were later given a physical basis with the identification of chromosomes, cellular structures that contain the genes that control inherited traits. To understand autosomal dominant inheritance, as well as other inheritance patterns, it is important to review some essential properties of chromosomes and genes and the rules governing their distribution in the process of sexual reproduction.

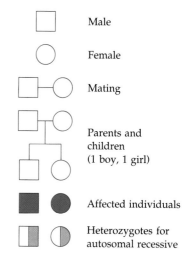

Some standard symbols used in depicting pedigrees.

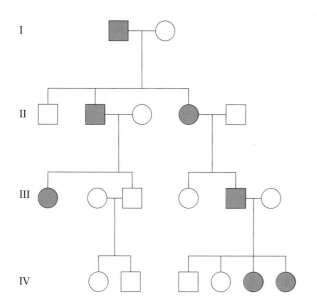

Transmission of Huntington's disease over four generations, illustrating the pattern of autosomal dominant inheritance.

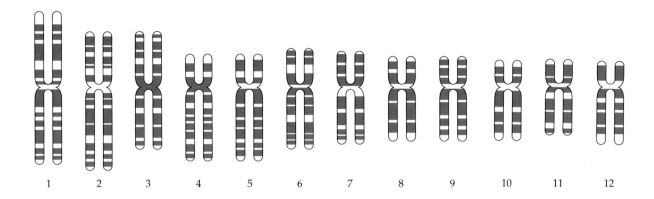

Human chromosomes. The drawings illustrate the characteristic sizes and shapes of the 22 autosomes and the 2 sex chromosomes, as well as the banding patterns observed when they are reacted with a stain called Giemsa. These chromosomes were collected from cells midway through the process of cell division, after each chromosome had duplicated. The two copies are held together at a point of attachment called the centromere. The largest chromosome (1) contains about 8 percent of the human genome.

Chromosomes and Heredity

At the beginning of the twentieth century, it became clear that the genes, whose existence Mendel had inferred, were contained in the nucleus of cells on structures called chromosomes. All normal human somatic cells (that is, all cells of the body other than sex cells) contain duplicate sets of 22 different chromosomes, called autosomes. Since one member of each pair of autosomes is derived from the mother and the other from the father, the two members of the pair are not identical and thus are referred to as being homologous (i.e., like but not identical). An additional set of nonhomologous chromosomes, the sex chromosomes X and Y, bring our full complement up to 23 pairs. Unlike autosomes, the sex chromosomes are unequally distributed in males and females. A female has two X and no Y, and a male has one X and one Y. This unequal distribution, which determines gender, is also responsible for a pattern of inheritance that is sex linked and will be considered later.

Genes are not distributed randomly within the chromosome pool. Instead, every chromosome contains particular genes arranged in a specific linear order, with each gene located at an identifiable position, called its locus, on a particular chromosome. Some genes (at the same locus) may exist in two or more alternative forms, called alleles. In the case of the gene that controls seed color in garden peas, one allele produces yellow color and the other produces green color. The gene in garden peas that controls the texture of seeds is located on a different chromosome than the gene for color. Again there are two alleles at the same locus, one generating a

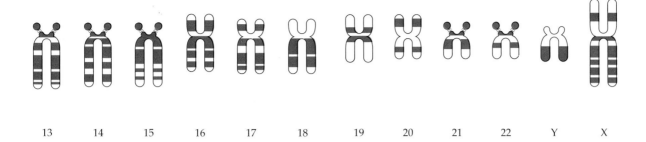

| 13 | 14 | 15 | 16 | 17 | 18 | 19 | 20 | 21 | 22 | Y | X |

smooth coat and the other a wrinkled coat. It is the separation of the genes for seed color and texture on different chromosomes that accounts for Mendel's seminal observation that these traits could be transmitted independently to a second generation of plants, yielding yellow peas or green peas either of which could be smooth or wrinkled.

The function of sexual reproduction is, in fact, to generate offspring with novel mixtures of genes. This is achieved through the production of sex cells, or gametes (that is, eggs and sperm). In the cell division that produces gametes, homologous chromosomes separate so that each gamete has half the autosomes. When gametes combine during fertilization, new combinations are generated. What ensures the diversity of the progeny is that the two members of each pair of chromosomes are independently assorted. This means that if there were only three chromosomes, as in the figure on the following page, we would be able to generate 2^3 chromosome combinations in our gametes. Since we have 22 autosomal pairs and a pair of sex chromosomes, we can each generate 2^{23} gamete variants.

Still greater diversity results from yet another mechanism, called crossing over, which occurs during gamete formation. In this process parts of homologous chromosomes are exchanged. In the example in the figure on page 27 only a single crossover is shown. Actually each pair of human chromosomes undergoes, on the average, more than two crossovers during gamete formation. Crossing over is of interest not only because it vastly increases gamete diversity but also because it helps geneticists to determine the relative locations of two genes that are both on the same chromosome, since genes that are close together are less likely to be separated by the essentially random breaks that occur in crossing over.

Independent assortment of chromosomes in the formation of sex cells.

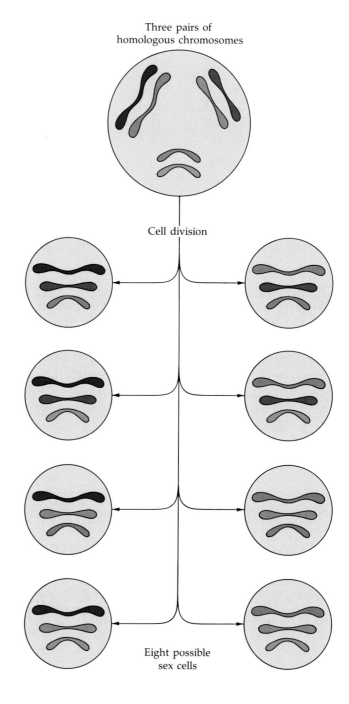

Three pairs of homologous chromosomes

Cell division

Eight possible sex cells

Chapter 2

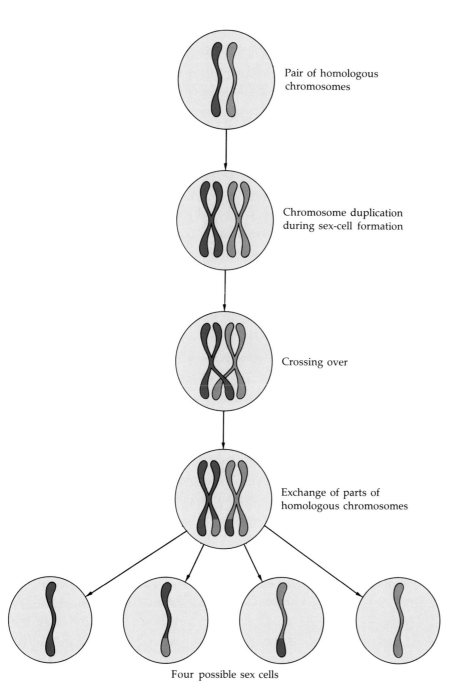

Pair of homologous chromosomes

Chromosome duplication during sex-cell formation

Crossing over

Exchange of parts of homologous chromosomes

Four possible sex cells

Chromosomal crossing over during sex-cell formation. Following duplication, homologous chromosomes come together in pairs. Breaks may occur at identical sites on the two chromosomes, allowing homologous pieces to be exchanged.

Autosomal dominant inheritance. The persons designated by pink boxes express the trait, in this case Huntington's disease.

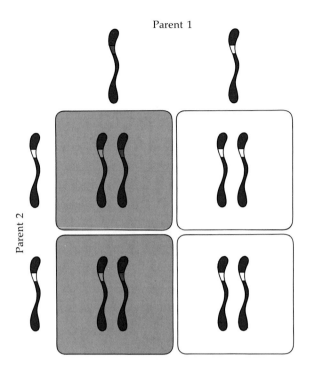

Knowing of the existence of chromosomes and their distribution during sexual reproduction makes it easy to infer what must be happening in autosomal dominant inheritance. To generate this pattern one allele must dominate the other, so that the phenotype of a heterozygote (with one copy of the dominant and one copy of the recessive allele) always reflects the trait dictated by the dominant rather than the recessive allele. Only a homozygote with two recessive alleles can express the recessive phenotype. Because of its dominance, half the children (on average) of a parent with Huntington's disease will not only inherit the abnormal allele (which is located on human chromosome 4) but will also, eventually, express the symptoms.

Besides autosomal dominant inheritance, there are two other major inheritance patterns: autosomal recessive inheritance and X-linked inheritance. These patterns are illustrated by two other human diseases that, like Huntington's disease, have characteristic and profound behavioral manifestations. Autosomal recessive inheritance is exemplified by phenylketonuria and X-linked inheritance by Lesch-Nyhan syndrome.

Phenylketonuria: Autosomal Recessive Inheritance

Phenylketonuria, or PKU, is a common genetic cause of mental retardation, affecting about one person in every 15,000 in northern European populations. Children with PKU are normal at birth, but if the condition is not treated, they will go on to develop symptoms that include small heads, irritability, and severe intellectual impairment. To express the disorder, a person must have two copies of the abnormal gene. This is the formal property that defines autosomal recessive inheritance. Many more people carry only one abnormal copy and have no symptoms.

The clue that helped identify the physical cause of phenylketonuria was a peculiar odor in the urine of affected children. Chemical analysis of the urine connected the odor to abnormally high concentrations of excreted

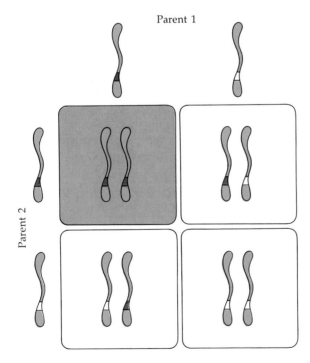

Autosomal recessive inheritance. The person designated by the pink box expresses the trait, in this case PKU.

Metabolism of phenylalanine. Normally phenylalanine is converted to tyrosine, which is used by the body for many purposes. However, in people with PKU, the enzyme phenylalanine hydroxylase, which catalyzes this conversion, is defective. As a result, phenylalanine builds up to toxic levels in the blood. Some of the phenylalanine is also degraded to phenylpyruvic acid by a scarce alternative enzyme. Although phenylpyruvic acid is normally a minor product, it becomes a major one in PKU because the pathway to tyrosine is blocked.

Phenylalanine hydroxylase

Hydroxyl group

NH_2

$CH_2-C-COOH$

H

Phenylalanine

NH_2

HO $CH_2-C-COOH$

H

Tyrosine

Alternative enzyme

O

$CH_2-C-COOH$

Phenylpyruvic acid

phenylketones, which are metabolic by-products of the amino acid phenylalanine, a component of dietary protein. Were phenylketones odorless, the cause of phenylketonuria might have remained a mystery for many years since there would have been no obvious lead to the underlying problem.

Subsequent work has demonstrated that phenylketones accumulate throughout the body because of a block in the normal metabolic conversion of phenylalanine to another amino acid, tyrosine. The cause of this block—and the cause of PKU—turned out to be a deficit in the enzyme phenylalanine hydroxylase, a protein in human cells that catalyzes the addition of a hydroxyl group (—OH) to phenylalanine to yield tyrosine. Because the enzyme is markedly impaired in affected individuals, large amounts of phenylalanine accumulate and some is degraded to phenylketones. The extremely high blood concentration of phenylalanine is believed to be primarily responsible for PKU mental retardation, but the details of the biochemical mechanisms that result in defective maturation of the developing brain are not yet known.

PKU infants can be easily detected by a simple test that measures the elevated concentration of phenylalanine in their blood. Fortunately, in the case of PKU, easy detection can be coupled with a practical remedy. Since the ultimate source of the toxic blood levels of phenylalanine is dietary protein, mental retardation may be prevented by restricting protein intake. The screening of all newborns for blood phenylalanine and the prescription of appropriate low-protein diets has markedly reduced the incidence of this form of mental retardation.

That a dietary change can influence the expression of a genetic abnormality is a lesson worth pondering, because it underscores the interaction

HEREDITY
(defective genes for
phenylalanine hydroxylase)

High blood levels
of phenylalanine → Abnormal
brain
development
in infancy
and childhood → Mental
retardation

ENVIRONMENT
(eating proteins, which are
rich in phenylalanine)

Heredity and environment are
both necessary in order for mental retardation to develop in people with PKU.

between heredity and environment. In this instance, the environmental
factor—that is, the amount of phenylalanine ingested—is clearly as important as the abnormal gene. In the case of other mental illnesses based on
genetic predispositions, relevant environmental factors may be more difficult to identify or define, but they may be equally significant nevertheless.

Transmission of phenylketonuria also demonstrates a pattern of inheritance that might initially seem puzzling: a lack of expression of the trait in
either the parents or the offspring of an affected individual. As can be seen
in the pedigree below, the pattern of autosomal recessive inheritance is
"horizontal," in that affected individuals tend to be limited to a single
sibship without representation of the disease in the preceding or succeeding generation. This contrasts strikingly with autosomal dominant inheritance, which is transmitted "vertically" from one generation to the next.

The locus of the gene that controls production of the enzyme phenylalanine hydroxylase is on chromosome 12. The normal allele is responsible

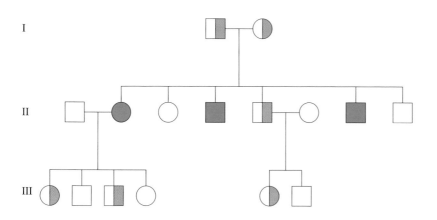

The appearance of PKU in generation II of a pedigree illustrating
the pattern of autosomal recessive
inheritance. Those people in each
generation who have only one
copy of the abnormal gene show
no signs of illness.

for the formation of normal phenylalanine hydroxylase, whereas the mutant allele produces an inactive form of the enzyme. How genes control enzyme structure will be considered in Chapter 3. For our present purposes, it is necessary only to recognize that a single normal allele is sufficient to produce enough active enzyme to support adequate, albeit diminished, conversion of phenylalanine to tyrosine. Therefore, a person who is heterozygous for this gene—that is, who carries one normal allele and one mutant allele—appears normal. Only a person with an abnormal allele on both chromosomes—that is, who is homozygous for the mutant allele—manifests the disease.

Since the mutant allele responsible for PKU tends to be quite rare in human populations, the probability that two people carrying it will mate is not high. The probability is increased if the couple are genetically related since both might have inherited the mutant allele from a common ancestor. For this reason, autosomal recessive diseases tend to be found more commonly in matings between close relatives.

Lesch-Nyhan Syndrome: X-Linked Inheritance

A third inheritance pattern is exemplified by Lesch-Nyhan syndrome. Although less prevalent than phenylketonuria, it too is a fairly common form of hereditary mental retardation. This disorder is caused by a mutant gene located on the X chromosome.

As with phenylketonuria, the relevant gene controls production of an enzyme. In this case the enzyme is hypoxanthine guanine phosphoribosyltransferase, which participates in the metabolism of purines, essential body constituents. Affected individuals show severe mental retardation, as well as other behavioral abnormalities, including a bizarre pattern of self-mutilation, especially finger biting, that results in great pain and deformity.

Implication of the X chromosome in the transmission of Lesch-Nyhan syndrome is indicated by two findings: only males are affected, and sons inherit the disorder from their unaffected mothers but not from their fathers. The latter pattern (which sounds a bit like a riddle) becomes comprehensible if we recall that males have only one X chromosome, which they always receive from their mother. Females have two X chromosomes, one from each parent. Consider then the children of a father who is normal and a mother with one X chromosome that contains the mutant allele. Half

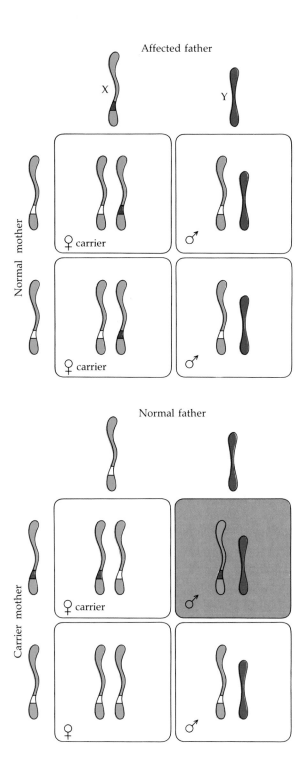

Sex-linked inheritance. The person designated by the pink box expresses the trait, in this case Lesch-Nyhan syndrome.

Sex-influenced inheritance of male pattern baldness over four generations. Whereas either parent may transmit this trait, male sex hormones are required for its expression.

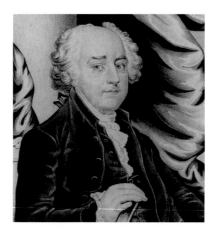

John Adams (1735–1826), second president of the United States.

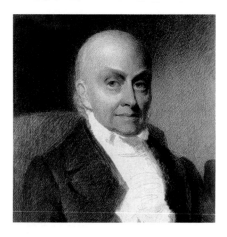

John Quincy Adams (1767–1848), sixth president of the United States.

of the male children would inherit the mother's abnormal X chromosome and hence the disease. In contrast, all of the daughters resulting from this marriage would have a normal phenotype even though they too have a 50 percent chance of receiving the X chromosome with the mutant allele. Their protection resides in the X chromosome that they receive from their father, which would provide sufficient amounts of the critical enzyme to allow normal brain development. However, half of the daughters would be heterozygote carriers who would, in turn, transmit the disorder to half of their sons.

Lesch-Nyhan syndrome is not the only X-linked form of hereditary mental retardation. Another, called fragile X syndrome, is also caused by an abnormality in a gene on the X chromosome. The gene is called FMR-1 (for "fragile X mental retardation-1"). The abnormality is associated both with breakage of the X chromosome within the FMR-1 locus (the basis for the designation "fragile") and with abnormal brain development that results in poor intellectual functioning. How this particular gene exerts its effects on the brain has not yet been determined.

Sex-linked inheritance involving the X chromosome must be distinguished from an important but distinct phenomenon called sex-influenced inheritance. A familiar example is male pattern baldness. This is an autosomal dominant trait (in that heterozygotes can express it) transmitted both by males and females; but it affects only males because expression of the abnormal allele depends on male sex hormones. In contrast, hormonally normal females with either one or two copies of the abnormal allele will have a full head of hair.

Chapter 2

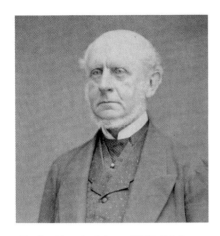

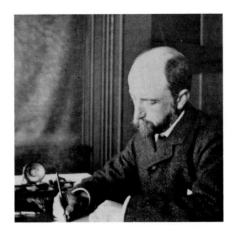

Charles Francis Adams (1807–1886), diplomat.

Henry Adams (1838–1918), historian.

Sex-influenced inheritance is worth noting because a number of psychiatric disorders are expressed in different ways and to different extents in males and females. For example, schizophrenia tends to begin much earlier in males, and females have a much higher incidence of major depression and certain anxiety disorders. Whether these differences reflect the direct influence of sex hormones on biological aspects of brain function, or the more indirect psychological influence of gender, is at present unknown.

Transferring a Complex Behavior with a Single Gene

So far we have discussed only hereditary behavioral diseases that involve major brain dysfunction. It is easy to understand how genetic abnormalities that produce obvious and extensive brain damage can give rise to mental symptoms. But the idea that individual genes might influence specific normal behaviors, without inducing gross brain changes, may be more difficult to accept.

Nevertheless, there are examples of the influence of single genes on complex behavior, without obvious effects on brain structure. The most convincing are seen in lower organisms, which have relatively simple nervous systems and behavioral repertoires. Insects, for example, are highly

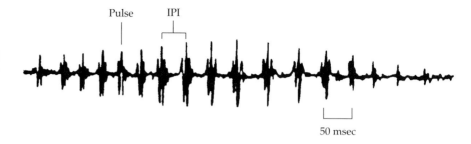

Pulse   IPI

50 msec

Audio recording of wing vibrations in the courtship song of *D. melanogaster* males. One feature of the song is the interpulse interval (IPI). This interval undergoes systematic variation. The period of the variation can be calculated.

programmed creatures. Because of their short life spans, it is more efficient for their behavior to be primarily controlled by genetic factors than by learning. In contrast, human behavior is designed to be influenced by experience and is less dependent on an inflexible genetic program.

A particularly good example of how a complex behavior can be controlled by a single gene is provided by the inheritance of the species-specific courtship songs of male fruit flies, genus *Drosophila*. The songs are produced by intermittent pulses of wing vibrations, which generate sounds that appeal to females of the same species and lead to mating. One critical aspect of these courtship songs is a property of the oscillation of interpulse intervals, here called the song-burst period. In normal *Drosophila melanogaster*, the fly species most frequently used for genetic experiments, this period tends to be about 60 seconds.

Over the past two decades, it has been shown that single-gene mutations in *D. melanogaster* have several effects on rhythmic behavior. Initially, Ronald Konopka and Seymour Benzer at the California Institute of Technology showed that individuals carrying the mutant gene manifested altered daily activity rhythms. (Like us, normal fruit flies have a periodicity of about 24 hours.) Subsequently, Jeffrey Hall and colleagues at Brandeis University found that these mutants also displayed different rhythmic properties in their courtship song-burst periods. For example, some mutants had unusually short daily activity periods of about 19 hours as well as short song-burst periods of about 30 seconds. Other mutants had unusually long daily activity periods of about 28 hours and song-burst periods of about 90 seconds. Still others had arrhythmic daily activity and song-burst periods. In each case, the unusual periods were transmitted to offspring in a pattern suggesting that they were due to mutations of a single gene on the X chromosome. The existence of these mutants, coupled with extensive knowledge of the genetic organization of *Drosophila* and excellent techniques for gene identification, led to the isolation of this gene, called *per* (for "period"). By studying the structure of the mutant genes (according to principles discussed in Chapter 3), researchers were able to correlate different structural changes in *per* with the different rhythms.

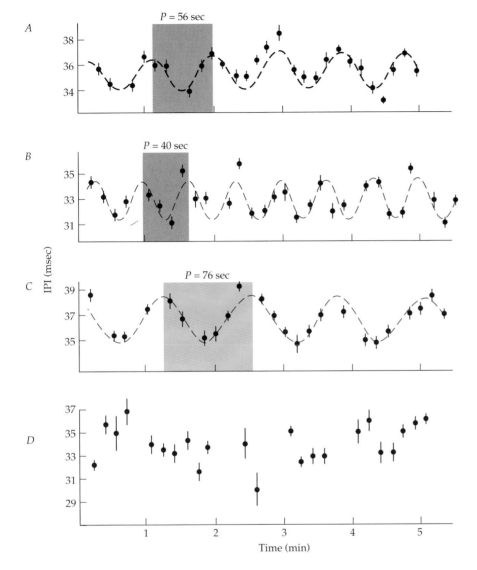

Song-burst patterns of a normal *Drosophila* male *(A)* and three types of mutants displaying short *(B)*, long *(C)*, and irregular *(D)* periods.

This information also made possible the isolation of the corresponding normal gene from another fruit fly species, *Drosophila simulans*, which has a normal courtship song period of 30 to 40 seconds. By comparing differences in the structure of the *per* genes of the two species, researchers could draw additional inferences about which parts of the gene control the behavioral rhythms. Even more remarkable, gene transfer experiments have been successfully performed, also in Hall's laboratory. For example, *per* genes from *D. simulans* have been introduced into arrhythmic mutants of *D. melanogaster*. The resultant genetically engineered *D. melanogaster* showed rhythmic courtship behavior with the song-burst period characteristic of *D. simulans*. When the same arrhythmic mutants were given normal *per* genes from *D. melanogaster*, the courtship song they expressed was also characteristic of the donor species. These stunning experiments prove that a specific behavior can be transmitted by a single gene.

Like the genes involved in PKU and Lesch-Nyhan syndrome, the *per* gene was found to direct the formation of a specific body protein. This finding led to the identification of a similar protein, which also appears to play a role in body rhythms, in several mammalian species. Although the chemical structure of the *per* gene protein was readily determined by means of well-established techniques (touched on in Chapter 3), the cellular mechanism by which it controls periodic behaviors in the fruit fly has not yet been elucidated. In fact, there is nothing about the chemical structure of the protein to suggest that *per* would have a behavioral effect, since it does not resemble proteins known to influence nervous system function.

The studies of *per* illustrate the great power of a genetic approach that begins with observation of a mutant phenotype (abnormal rhythms) and proceeds to identification of the relevant gene and the body protein it is responsible for, thereby setting the stage for new insights into the way in which this previously unknown protein controls behavior. Eventually, comparable success may be achieved with Huntington's disease; at present, we know only the approximate location of the relevant gene, not its precise location or its chemical structure. A more detailed understanding of this and other genes that play a role in human mental illness may reveal that they too are responsible for hitherto unknown brain proteins and cellular mechanisms.

Some Behavioral Traits Are Controlled by Multiple Genes

All the examples considered so far illustrate how single genes can have profound effects on behavior. It is probable, however, that most human behavioral traits, including variants of psychiatric interest, are influenced by the concerted action of a number of genes, which are transferred from generation to generation by a process called polygenic inheritance.

Dogs bred for both appearance and behavioral traits.

Our appreciation of polygenic inheritance of behavioral traits is based largely on animal studies. Much of the classic work was done centuries ago by animal breeders. These individuals had no knowledge of genes or chromosomes; nevertheless, they found that they could develop distinct breeds within a given species by gradually selecting for certain desired features, such as color, size, or behavior. A great deal of the animal work to date has been done with dogs. There are many breeds, each characterized not only by a specific appearance but also by behavioral traits. Some breeds can be readily trained to track or point to prey, others to herd sheep. Some are by nature placid and cuddly, whereas others are more high-strung, or territorial, or aggressive. Such traits are maintained by inbreeding and lost by interbreeding, in patterns suggesting that multiple genes are involved.

Although dogs demonstrate the inherited nature of behavioral propensities very convincingly, they are not optimal subjects for formal research on mammalian behavioral inheritance. For experimental purposes, mice have a number of advantages over dogs. First, their period of gestation is relatively short, about three weeks, and they reach sexual maturity within about two months after birth. Thus, several generations can be bred in a single year, facilitating multigenerational studies. Mice are also small and relatively easy to maintain. These same characteristics also make them particularly useful subjects for studies of general properties of mammalian inheritance. As a result of such studies, a growing number of mouse genes can now be precisely located on their chromosomes, and this body of information can help researchers to localize and identify new genes with behavioral effects.

Mouse-breeding studies have yielded strong evidence for multiple-gene influences on behavior. One trait that has been examined in detail by J. C. DeFries and colleagues at the University of Colorado, called open-field behavior, is a measure of reaction to being placed in a large space (an "open field") under stressful circumstances. The reaction is assessed experimentally when individual mice are placed in a brightly illuminated and unfamiliar box and then their exploratory movements over a given period are measured with an automatic sensing device. Some mice find the experience very stressful and may freeze or huddle in a corner. Such mice are considered to be highly "emotional" (to use a loose term). In contrast, mice that explore the box confidently are considered less emotional. Whatever the mice are actually feeling, the amount of open-field activity is what is recorded.

The degree of emotionality in mice is under the control of multiple genes, as evidenced by progressive selective breeding of mice with relatively high and relatively low open-field scores over 30 generations. Repetitive mating of the most emotional or the least emotional siblings of a given generation resulted in the gradual selection of animals with far higher or far lower open-field activity than the ancestral stock. The fact that the divergence was progressive over many generations indicates that multiple genes are operative in controlling the behavior being selected. In single-gene inheritance, the trait in question is either expressed or absent in a given individual. In the case of open-field activity, in contrast, there is a gradual trend toward greater or lesser emotionality in a given population, with extremely variant animals appearing only after many generations of breeding. It is not a simple case of one gene negating the effect of an alternative allele, but of multiple genes acting together to produce an evolving phenotype.

There is reason to believe that complex human personality traits are also influenced by the concerted action of a number of particular genes. This is, of course, more difficult to study in humans than in mice, since human mating is determined by caprice rather than experimental design. One approach is to compare personality traits, measured by elaborate formal questionnaires, in people with different degrees of genetic identity.

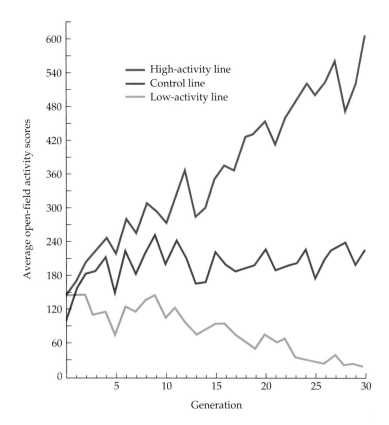

Average open-field activity scores of three lines of mice bred over 30 generations. One line was selected by mating mice with high open-field activity and another by mating mice with low open-field activity. A third line was randomly mated to serve as a control.

Traits measured in such studies include "social potency" (strives to be a leader), "harm avoidance" (low tendency to risk taking), "traditionalism" (follows rules and authority), and "sense of well-being." Comparisons are made between unrelated people, siblings, fraternal twins, and identical twins. Siblings and fraternal twins share half their genes, whereas identical twins, obviously, share all genes.

The consistent finding of these studies is that identical twins are far more similar than fraternal twins or siblings. Similarity can be expressed as a formal statistical correlation, in which the lack of any correlation, as would be expected in randomly selected individuals, would be 0, and a perfect correlation would be 1.0. The overall result of twin studies comparing various personality traits is that fraternal twins have a correlation of about 0.25, whereas identical twins have a correlation of about 0.50.

Of course, identical twins generally live in very similar environments, and this may be the cause of their shared personality traits. One argument against this explanation is that fraternal twins are also raised together yet

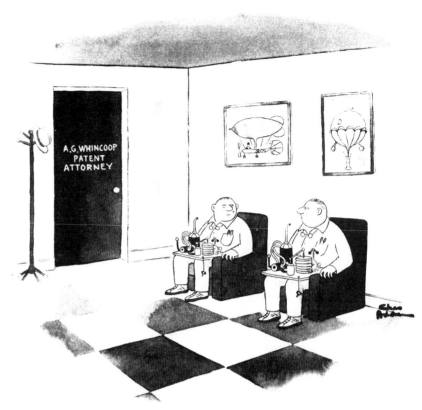

Separated at birth, the Mallifert twins meet accidentally.

show a lower correlation. An even more striking argument derives from the body of evidence accumulated by a group of psychologists at the University of Minnesota, including Thomas Bouchard, David Lykken, and Auke Tellegen, that 44 pairs of identical twins reared apart since an early age were as similar in personality traits as identical twins reared together. In both the pairs reared together and those reared apart, the trait correlations were about 0.50. What is particularly remarkable about this finding is that it challenges assumptions that being raised in the same family has much to do with personality. Were that true, identical twins reared in the same family should be even more similar than those reared apart. In fact, the surprising conclusion of this study is that the considerable similarities in the personalities of identical twins seem to be completely attributable to their genes. It is also noteworthy, however, that for both the separated and unseparated pairs of identical twins, correlations are 0.5, not 1.0. Therefore, factors other than genes (i.e., environmental factors) contribute to personality. These factors could be psychological, biological, or both.

The Challenge of Polygenic Inheritance
and Genetic Heterogeneity

The early examples in this chapter make behavioral genetics look both simple and practical. This is especially true of PKU. Only one gene is involved; and once the gene was identified, an effective remedy quickly followed. It is probable, however, that the polygenic inheritance of emotionality in mice is a better model not only for other complex behavioral traits but also for many common psychiatric disorders. If this is so, discovery of the relevant genes promises to be a challenging problem since tracking down multiple genes that act together to produce a particular phenotype requires far more effort than identifying a single gene. It is encouraging, however, that researchers have already had some success in identifying several genes that act together to produce diabetes in human beings as well as several others that produce hypertension in mice.

Another phenomenon, called genetic heterogeneity, also complicates the search for genes responsible for a particular psychiatric disorder. The meaning of genetic heterogeneity is that the same general phenotype, such as depression or schizophrenia, may result from the action of different abnormal genes (either single or multiple). We have already seen examples of this in the case of another general phenotype, mental retardation, which can be caused by abnormalities in the gene responsible for PKU, the gene responsible for Lesch-Nyhan syndrome, or the gene responsible for fragile X syndrome.

One way to try to sidestep the problem of genetic heterogeneity is to focus attention on large families with many affected members. One can tentatively assume that because all of the affected members are related, they all have not only the same phenotype but also the same genetic disorder, possibly derived from a single ancestor. Since there are many affected members as well as many unaffected members, there should be enough data points to permit statistically reliable estimates of the relationship between a particular gene and the behavior in question.

In future chapters, we will consider the role of inheritance in psychiatric disorders. But before these issues are addressed, it is important to review briefly the chemical nature of the genetic material and our current understanding of the ways in which genes control the structure and functioning of nerve cells and the brain. This will make possible a deeper understanding of how abnormal genes can be identified and of the ways genes affect behavior.

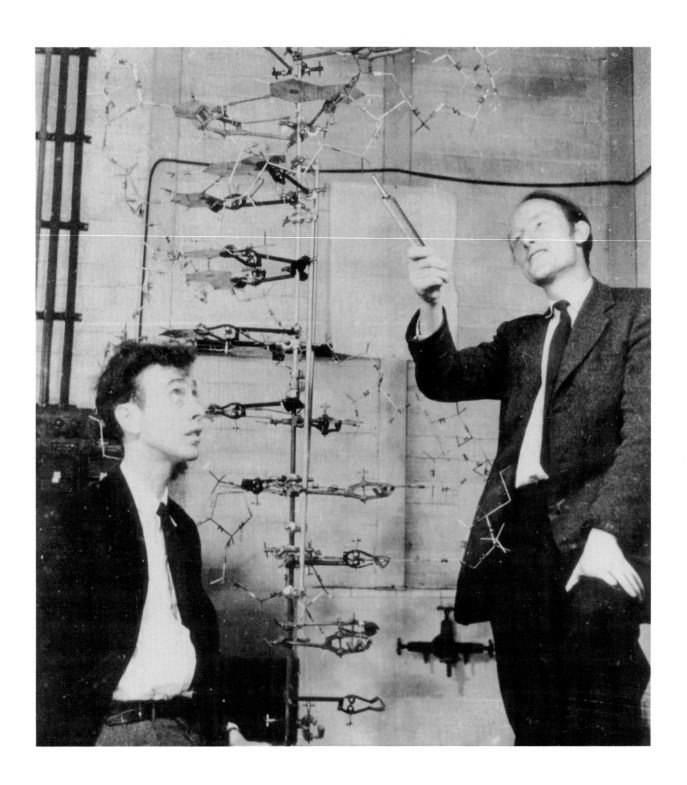

3

HOW GENES WORK

The genetic principles described in the preceding chapter provide only a preliminary foundation for understanding inherited propensities to certain behaviors. A fuller appreciation requires that we review how the genes, the fundamental units of heredity, express their innate messages via a several-stage process that culminates in synthesis of proteins. For it is specific brain proteins, finally, that control the cellular functions underlying behavior; if only one of these proteins is abnormal, it may cause or predispose to specific mental illness. The purpose of this chapter is to provide the reader with the biological background needed to grasp how genes and proteins exert their behavioral effects.

This may be more than some readers bargained for. It's one thing to have to struggle through a chapter on the general principles of heredity, since that does seem to have some direct bearing on behavior. But is it

OPPOSITE: James Watson (1928–) with Francis Crick (1916–), who is pointing at their 1953 model of DNA.

really necessary to deal with molecules in order to appreciate psychiatry? The reason it is, is that molecules are the chemical machinery of our brains, so that to study them is to study the actual brain components involved in feeling and remembering, instead of contemplating these processes only at a high level of abstraction.

This is not to say that our current knowledge of the brain is up to the challenge of explaining behavior. We are in fact very far from this goal. But readers who wish to think seriously about what inheritance of mental illness means and how drugs are used to treat it will find their understanding deepened by the fundamental information presented in this chapter.

DNA, *the Genetic Material*

Genes are composed of deoxyribonucleic acid, a very long molecular chain more commonly referred to by its abbreviation, DNA. DNA is composed of smaller molecular building blocks called nucleotides, each consisting of a phosphate, a sugar (deoxyribose), and one of four other components: adenine (A), guanine (G), thymine (T), or cytosine (C)—the so-called bases. The bases are the essential message-carrying units of DNA. Linked together by strong chemical bonds between the sugar-phosphates, the nucleotides form long chains, or polymers, with the bases strung along them like beads. Given the biological complexity it gives rise to, our entire hereditary legacy comprises a remarkably small number of elements: 23 DNA molecules from each parent (one DNA molecule per chromosome), which together contain about 100,000 different genes. Each gene contains from a few thousand to several hundred thousand nucleotides. Our entire genome is only three billion nucleotides long.

The central role of DNA in the transfer of hereditary information depends on an intrinsic property of its four constituent bases. Each base is so constituted that it tends to associate, by specific chemical bonds, with a particular one of the other bases, to which it is said to be complementary. Adenine and thymine are mutually complementary, as are guanine and cytosine.

One result of DNA base pairing is the generation of a stable chemical structure made up of two complementary chains of nucleotides, the famous DNA double helix first described in 1953 by James Watson and Fran-

Complementary base pairing of A with T and G with C by means of hydrogen bonds.

cis Crick, then working at Cambridge University. In elucidating the molecular structure of DNA, Watson and Crick reached the seminal conclusion that base pairing not only serves to hold DNA together but also underlies DNA replication. During replication, the two chains of the double helix separate, and each acts as a template for the formation of a new companion chain. Free nucleotides bind with the exposed complementary bases in the template strands and are then linked together by an enzyme, DNA polymerase, to make two new complementary chains—and one complete replica of the double helix. The sequence of base pairs in the original DNA molecule is duplicated exactly, so that the genetic information it carries can be transmitted from one cell to its descendants. Obviously this replication must be error-free, since a skip or a base substitution will be copied and transmitted to the succeeding cell generations. As we have already seen, changes of this kind, called mutations, can be the culprits in genetic diseases, including psychiatric disorders.

Base pairing of two DNA chains. The sugar-phosphate backbones are held together by covalent bonds that join each phosphate group to the 5′ carbon of one deoxyribose and the 3′ carbon of the next.

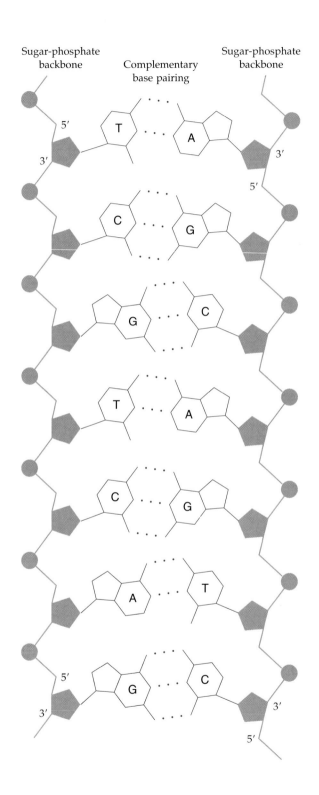

Sugar-phosphate backbone

Complementary base pairing

Sugar-phosphate backbone

Translating the Genetic Code

DNA transmits the information that determines the structure of the major cellular constituents, the proteins, by an ordered series of steps beginning with the construction of an intermediary molecule called messenger RNA (abbreviated mRNA). Messenger RNA carries the genetic messages from the nucleus, where DNA resides, to the machinery that makes proteins in the cytoplasm of the cell. Like DNA, mRNAs are polymers of linked nucleotides; unlike DNA, however, they are made up of single-stranded nucleotide chains. Messenger RNAs also differ from DNA in that the base thymine is replaced by uracil (U) (which, like T, is complementary to A), and the constituent sugar is ribose rather than deoxyribose.

The specific structure of individual messenger RNA molecules is determined by complementary base pairing on a DNA template, with the aid of the enzyme RNA polymerase. In contrast to DNA replication, in which the entire template strands of a chromosome, consisting of many millions of nucleotides, are replicated from beginning to end, mRNA synthesis is confined to a single gene, and gives rise to a product that generally contains only a few thousand nucleotides. Furthermore, mRNAs are generated from only one strand of the double helix, as is shown in the diagram below. Instructions for starting and stopping RNA synthesis are encoded in short sequences of nucleotides within the DNA. The process of polymerizing an mRNA from a gene, called transcription, is controlled by a team of

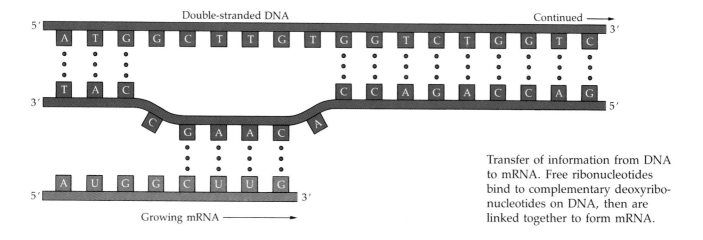

Transfer of information from DNA to mRNA. Free ribonucleotides bind to complementary deoxyribonucleotides on DNA, then are linked together to form mRNA.

regulatory proteins known as transcription factors, which must associate with RNA polymerase and DNA for mRNA synthesis to proceed. Transcription factors may be influenced by internal developmental or external environmental cues in ways that affect mRNA synthesis, thus controlling the expression of specific genes.

By means of the nucleotide sequence imparted to it by DNA, an mRNA directs the synthesis of a specific protein. This process is different from the base pairing that yields DNA and mRNA. The four-letter language of nucleic acids must, in effect, be translated into the twenty-letter language of proteins. Each of the 20 different amino acids from which protein polymers are made is specified by a sequence of three consecutive nucleotides, called a codon. A codon with the base sequence UUU, for example, codes for the insertion of the amino acid phenylalanine into a growing protein, whereas AUG codes for the insertion of the amino acid methionine.

With only a four-base alphabet, the language potential of RNA might seem to be limited. But since the code is based on sequences of three nucleotides, this allows for 64 possible combinations, which could, in principle, direct the incorporation of as many as 64 different amino acids. Although only 20 amino acids are actually used to construct proteins, none of the 64 possibilities is wasted, because most amino acids are encoded by more

Amino Acids and Their Symbols

A	Ala	Alanine	M	Met	Methionine
C	Cys	Cysteine	N	Asn	Asparagine
D	Asp	Aspartic acid	P	Pro	Proline
E	Glu	Glutamic acid	Q	Gln	Glutamine
F	Phe	Phenylalanine	R	Arg	Arginine
G	Gly	Glycine	S	Ser	Serine
H	His	Histidine	T	Thr	Threonine
I	Ile	Isoleucine	V	Val	Valine
K	Lys	Lysine	W	Trp	Tryptophan
L	Leu	Leucine	Y	Tyr	Tyrosine

	Arg									Leu					Ser				Val	
	AGA									UUA					AGC					
	AGG									UUG					AGU					
GCA	CGA						GGA			CUA				CCA	UCA	ACA			GUA	
GCC	CGC						GGC		AUA	CUC				CCC	UCC	ACC				UAA
GCG	CGG	GAC	AAC	UGC	GAA	CAA	GGG	CAC	AUC	CUG	AAA		UUC	CCG	UCG	ACG		UAC	GUG	UAG
GCU	CGU	GAU	AAU	UGU	GAG	CAG	GGU	CAU	AUU	CUU	AAG	AUG	UUU	CCU	UCU	ACU	UGG	UAU	GUU	UGA
Ala	Arg	Asp	Asn	Cys	Glu	Gln	Gly	His	Ile	Leu	Lys	Met	Phe	Pro	Ser	Thr	Trp	Tyr	Val	stop
A	R	D	N	C	E	Q	G	H	I	L	K	M	F	P	S	T	W	Y	V	

than one codon. Of the 64 codons, 61 encode amino acids, whereas the remaining three, called stop codons, are used for another purpose—to signal termination of translation.

Messenger RNA translation does not occur by direct association of a codon with its amino acid; it requires a molecular adapter called a transfer RNA (tRNA). Transfer RNAs are a specialized group of RNA molecules, each of which is designed to bind to a specific codon in messenger RNA and to the amino acid it encodes. Each tRNA contains a three-nucleotide sequence, called an anticodon, that is complementary to a codon in mRNA. For each of the 20 amino acids, there are one or more specific enzymes that catalyze its linkage to the appropriate tRNA molecules. The amino acids coupled to tRNAs are ultimately transferred onto a growing chain that will, when its three-dimensional structure is established, function biologically as a protein.

Above: The genetic code. Sequences of three nucleotides in mRNA, called codons, direct the incorporation of particular amino acids during protein synthesis. Note that there is more than one codon for most amino acids.

Translation of mRNA into protein. The anticodon on a tRNA binds to a complementary codon on the mRNA, directing incorporation of the appropriate amino acid into the growing protein chain.

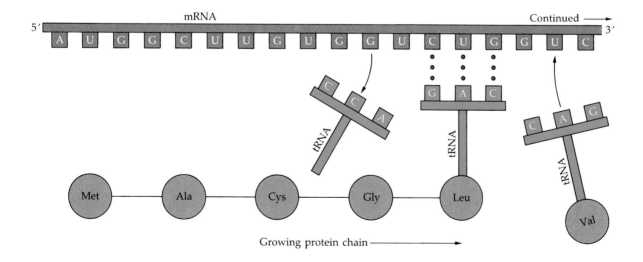

The Structure of Proteins

Whereas DNA is the ultimate repository of biological information, most of the functions that it directs are carried out by proteins. The 20 different amino acids each have special chemical characteristics that cause the proteins they are part of to fold and bend into particular three-dimensional shapes. For example, some amino acids are hydrophobic, which means that they prefer lipid environments to the water in body fluids and so tend to move to the inside of folded proteins. In contrast, other amino acids are hydrophilic, which means that they are attracted to water, and so tend to migrate to a protein's outer surface. Particular amino acids also have other important properties, such as positive or negative electric charge causing them to attract or repel each other, that also influence the final protein structure. Thus, the amino acid sequence of a protein dictates its form and, ultimately, its biological function.

The work of proteins depends on intermolecular binding with specific molecules called ligands (from the Latin *ligare*, "to bind"). Enzymes, such as those that catalyze the tRNA–amino acid linking just discussed, provide an example of ligand-specific binding, one ligand in this case being a particular amino acid. The enzyme contains a specifically configured binding site, which may be thought of as a groove whose shape and chemical properties are such that its specific ligand fits into it as a key fits into a lock. Individual proteins may have binding sites for more than one ligand: for

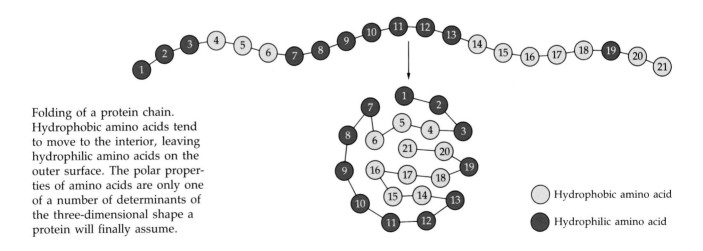

Folding of a protein chain. Hydrophobic amino acids tend to move to the interior, leaving hydrophilic amino acids on the outer surface. The polar properties of amino acids are only one of a number of determinants of the three-dimensional shape a protein will finally assume.

○ Hydrophobic amino acid

● Hydrophilic amino acid

Chapter 3

example, the enzymes that link amino acids to tRNA have specific sites for both a particular amino acid and a particular tRNA.

Although the shapes and the binding sites of proteins are specialized, they are not fixed. Some proteins (called allosteric, from the Greek words for "another" and "solid") are designed to alternate from an inactive to an active conformation. One of these conformations may be stabilized by the binding of a specialized ligand, such as a hormone or a neurotransmitter. There is, for example, a class of nerve-cell proteins that controls the opening and closing of channels for the passage of electrically charged particles in or out of the cell. The binding of an appropriate neurotransmitter stabilizes such proteins in a configuration that holds the channels open, whereas the release of the ligand allows the channels to close. Many aspects of neuronal excitation and synaptic transmission involve such reversible changes in protein shape, as we will see in the next chapter.

Protein functions may be modified not only by temporary ligand binding but also by more permanent changes in a protein's chemical structure. Such changes may involve coupling certain chemical residues to an amino acid in the protein chain by means of strong chemical bonds. Since these alterations occur after protein translation and are not directly controlled by the genetic code, they are called post-translational modifications.

Post-translational modifications to a protein's chemical structure are relatively stable. Formation or breakage of the strong chemical bonds involved requires the assistance of special enzymes. The new chemical structure tends to persist for seconds or minutes or longer, until terminated by enzyme action, in contrast with changes based on reversible ligand binding, which may last only fractions of a second and terminate with ligand

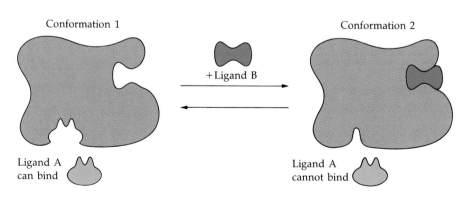

Conformation 1   + Ligand B   Conformation 2

Ligand A can bind

Ligand A cannot bind

An allosteric protein. The protein shown tends to assume a shape in which it binds a particular ligand, such as a neurotransmitter. However, should this protein bind another ligand, such as a natural regulatory molecule or a drug, at another specialized binding site, it is stabilized in a new shape that can no longer bind the first ligand. In other cases two ligands may augment each other's binding or exert still other effects that control the function of the protein.

Regulation of protein shape by phosphorylation. The protein shown tends to assume a shape that will bind a particular ligand, but its shape and binding ability are altered if a phosphate residue is covalently attached to a particular amino acid that forms part of its outer surface. When the phosphate is removed, the protein regains its original conformation and binding characteristics.

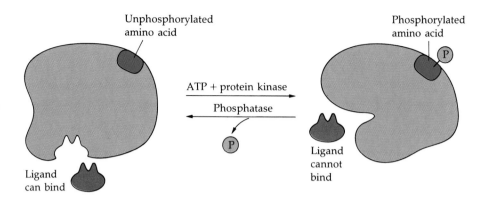

Unphosphorylated amino acid

Phosphorylated amino acid

ATP + protein kinase

Phosphatase

Ligand can bind

Ligand cannot bind

dissociation. The duration of a conformational change resulting either from ligand binding or from chemical modification defines the length of a protein's molecular memory and is critical for information processing in the nervous system. It may even underlie subjectively discernible behavioral memories.

An important class of post-translational modifications involves the addition of a phosphate residue to certain amino acids in a given protein; this is known as phosphorylation. A special class of enzymes called protein kinases has evolved, each of which is specialized to phosphorylate certain proteins. The ways a protein is phosphorylated are determined, in part, by the types of protein kinases that are expressed in the cells in which the protein resides, which is under stringent biological regulation.

The change in protein structure produced by phosphorylation can be reversed by the action of enzymes called phosphatases, which remove phosphate residues. The dephosphorylated protein then reverts to its original state. Many proteins that influence neuronal activity and behavior are regulated by phosphorylation and dephosphorylation, as we shall see in later chapters.

Selective Gene Expression

Only a fraction of our genes are dedicated to the basic cellular processes (e.g., respiration and metabolism) that are the indispensable housekeeping functions of life. Such genes are expressed in all cells and must be active at all times. In complex organisms, however, individual cells may express certain genes extensively while failing to express many others. Selective gene expression underlies all cellular specialization. Nowhere is this more apparent than in the brain, an organ composed of hundreds of different types of nerve cells, each of which has special properties defined by the unique mixture of proteins it expresses. Of the 100,000 different proteins encoded in the human genome, about a third are expressed *only* in the brain and appear to be specifically committed to its many complex functions.

To achieve differentiation, embryonic cells must contain a mechanism whereby specific genes are turned on or off at different stages in their development. This area of cell biology is currently under intensive investigation. An important component of this switching mechanism is the diverse array of transcription factors mentioned above. The control these regulatory proteins have over transcription of mRNA from individual genes helps determine the particular proteins that different classes of ma-

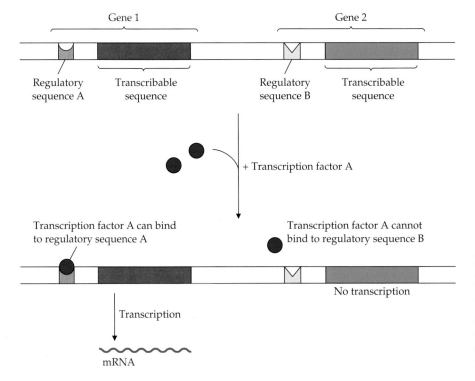

Gene 1

Gene 2

Regulatory sequence A

Transcribable sequence

Regulatory sequence B

Transcribable sequence

+ Transcription factor A

Transcription factor A can bind to regulatory sequence A

Transcription factor A cannot bind to regulatory sequence B

No transcription

Transcription

mRNA

Expression of the transcribable sequence of a gene is controlled by a transcription factor that binds to a specific regulatory sequence. In reality many transcription factors act in concert to control the expression of a particular gene.

ture neurons will express. These include neurotransmitters and receptor proteins, as well as surface proteins that influence the contacts neurons make with other neurons to form neuronal circuits.

Whereas some genetic regulatory processes are chiefly involved in establishing permanent characteristics of developing cells, others are concerned with reversible adaptive responses in mature cells. Examples of the latter are displayed in the body's response to intense stress, which may activate genes that help protect against danger. A major participant in the stress response is the adrenal cortex, which releases a class of steroid hormones called glucocorticoids into the bloodstream. The glucocorticoids circulate throughout the body, binding to a protein called the glucocorticoid receptor, which is expressed in many different types of cells. Such binding makes this receptor protein function as a transcription factor in these cells, triggering the expression of certain genes. The proteins synthesized as a result produce a complex series of changes in the body. Some enhance metabolic processes that favor alertness or defensive reactions; others suppress immune function or produce other undesirable effects that we associate with unremitting stress.

Critical Facts about Genes and Proteins

1. Nucleotides (with their four different bases) are the elemental building blocks of all genes.

2. The human genome consists of 3 billion nucleotides, which make up about 100,000 genes.

3. A single gene contains between a few thousand and several million nucleotides.

4. Part of each gene encodes a particular protein structure (some of the remainder is used for regulation).

5. Sequences of three bases (codons) code for each amino acid in proteins.

6. Twenty amino acids are the elemental building blocks of all proteins.

7. Most proteins contain between 100 and 1000 amino acids.

8. The amino-acid sequence of a protein determines its folding and its ultimate shape, which defines its function.

Emergent Complexity

It should be apparent from this brief overview that DNA encodes sufficient information to generate enormous biological complexity: linear sequences of its four constituent nucleotides ultimately direct the formation of 100,000 body proteins, each of which has special properties. From the interactions of this broad array of proteins—both with each other and with nucleic acids—elaborate cellular structures have evolved. One result has been the development of thinking and feeling organisms.

Understanding molecular genetics is, therefore, critical for understanding cognition and emotion. Although behavior may seem remote from complementary base pairing and protein conformation, the relevance of such molecular properties to both practical and theoretical matters in psychiatry will be evident throughout the remainder of this book. How such fundamental investigations have enriched our understanding of some of the brain proteins whose functions most immediately underlie behavior will be addressed in the next chapter.

Appendix: Applying Base Pairing to Genetic Diagnosis

The simple property of complementary base pairing is not only of theoretical interest. It is also central to a rapidly evolving DNA technology with which we now can directly examine the genetic structure of individual human beings in search of sequence variations that are correlated with specific disease states, including psychiatric disorders. The ultimate goal of this research is to find the abnormal genes that cause disease. One step along the way is to find where disease genes are located on particular chromosomes. The purpose of this appendix is to provide the interested reader with a brief introduction to the techniques that are being developed to achieve this goal.

Part of the new technology involves identifying short sequences of bases within the human genome and synthesizing segments of DNA that are complementary. Suppose, for example, that we determine that an individual gene, or other bit of human DNA, contains a run of nucleotides with the base sequence CCGCTATCGACTGAG and then chemically synthesize

Some Restriction Enzymes
and the Base Sequences They Cleave

BACTERIAL SOURCE	ENZYME	SEQUENCE
Escherichia coli	*Eco*RV	5′ . . . G A T|A T C . . . 3′ 3′ . . . C T A|T A G . . . 5′
Escherichia coli	*Eco*RI	5′ . . . G|A A T T C . . . 3′ 3′ . . . C T T A A|G . . . 5′
Haemophilus haemolyticus	*Hha*I	5′ . . . G C G|C . . . 3′ 3′ . . . C|G C G . . . 5′
Providencia stuarti	*Pst*I	5′ . . . C T G C A|G . . . 3′ 3′ . . . G A|C G T C . . . 5′

Facing page: Analyzing human DNA by Southern blotting. A sample of DNA is extracted from a person's cells and, in the case shown here, cleaved with one of five different restriction enzymes. The cleaved DNA is then applied to an agarose gel and electrophoretically separated by size. The DNA in the gel is then transferred to a nitrocellulose filter and allowed to hybridize with a radioactively labeled DNA probe. Hybridization specifically identifies the sequence that is complementary to the probe, even though it represents only a tiny amount of the total DNA on the filter. After unbound probe is washed off, the filter is applied to an X-ray film. The radioactivity in the remaining probe shows up as dark areas on the developed film (called an autoradiogram) that reveal the locations of the DNA complementary to the probe. Because the cleavage sites for the five different restriction enzymes used in this experiment are at different distances from the targeted DNA sequence, fragments of different sizes are generated, as reflected by the different distances of migration in each of the five lanes.

complementary DNA with the base sequence GGCGATAGCTGACTC. If the complementary fragment is introduced into a sample of native DNA, it will act as a probe by hybridizing (i.e., binding) to the gene in the native DNA that has the original sequence. The probe is made detectable by the addition of a radioactive label. If the probe comprises a long enough string of nucleotides, there will be only one sequence in the genome to which it will be perfectly complementary and thus hybridize.

In preparation for probe analysis it is necessary to break the very long strands of native DNA up into smaller pieces. This task is accomplished by a family of special enzymes (derived from bacteria) called restriction enzymes. Hundreds of different restriction enzymes are available. Each one recognizes a unique DNA sequence, generally four to eight bases long; it binds to the DNA at that location and cleaves it into smaller pieces. The length of the pieces ranges from a few hundred to a few thousand nucleotides; but the pattern of pieces that is generated is unique for each restriction enzyme, since this depends on the distribution of the specific sequence that the enzyme cleaves.

The chopped-up DNA is then applied to a thin slab of porous gel, and the fragments are separated, based on their length, by means of a procedure called gel electrophoresis. An electric current is run through the gel that causes the fragments to migrate down the gel, the shorter fragments traveling faster, and hence farther, from the starting position than the longer fragments. Simple inspection of the gel reveals a graduated series of

Chapter 3

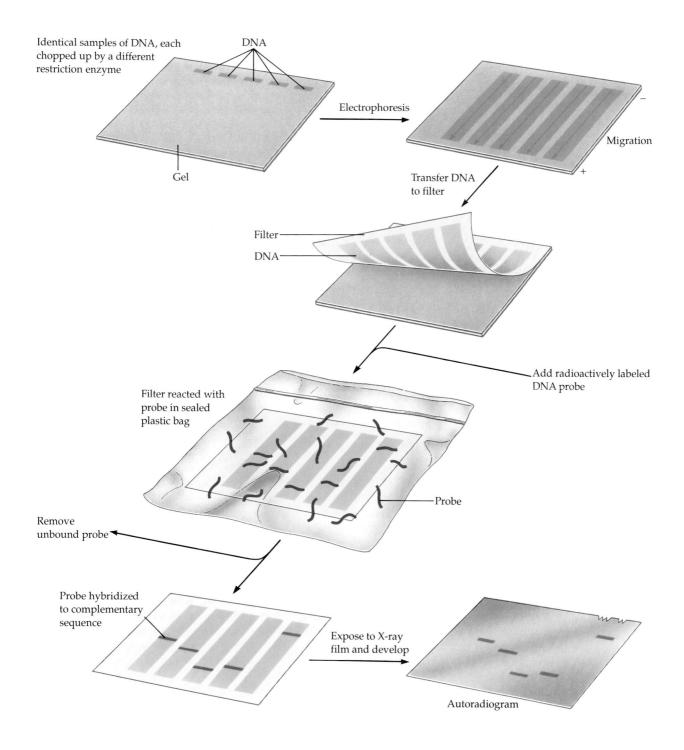

Identical samples of DNA, each chopped up by a different restriction enzyme

DNA

Gel

Electrophoresis

Migration

−

+

Transfer DNA to filter

Filter

DNA

Add radioactively labeled DNA probe

Filter reacted with probe in sealed plastic bag

Probe

Remove unbound probe

Probe hybridized to complementary sequence

Expose to X-ray film and develop

Autoradiogram

DNA fragments of different lengths. However, a smear containing fragments of every possible size is not in itself informative—we still do not know which size fragment contains the DNA sequence that is being sought. This is where base pairing comes in. The gel can be reacted with a radioactive probe that is complementary to that sequence. In practice, the electrophoresed DNA is first blotted onto a filter before it is reacted with a probe. The DNA that the probe binds is then detected by applying the filter to an X-ray film. The binding site of the radioactive probe shows up as darkening on the developed X-ray film. The entire procedure, introduced by E. M. Southern, is called Southern blotting.

One reason Southern blotting is such a valuable tool is that it can be used to detect a single base variation in the entire sequence of human DNA—either in the sequence complementary to the probe or in adjacent regions. Whereas some base variations may be responsible for genetic disorders, most of them have no functional consequences. In fact, all people carry innocuous sequence variations in their DNA; these occur at a rate of approximately one every thousand bases. Such variations are called polymorphisms (from the Greek, meaning "multiple forms") and are as insignificant to basic life processes as more obvious polymorphisms like eye color. Some polymorphisms occur in regions of DNA that are known recognition sites for specific restriction enzymes and thus can determine whether or not there is cleavage at those locations. Consequently, if Southern blotting is performed on the DNA of two individuals, one with a base variation at the recognition site, and the other without, different fragment lengths will be obtained. The variation in fragment length is called a restriction fragment length polymorphism (RFLP).

Like all DNA sequences, those encoding RFLPs are faithfully transmitted from parents to children, just as any other heritable trait is. One goal of human genetic research has been to develop probes that define specific locations on particular chromosomes and that are adjacent to polymorphic sequences in DNA called markers. The markers can then be used to localize disease genes that are near (or linked to) them in a particular chromosome, as in the diagram on the next page. By using probes for a series of several hundred polymorphic markers that have been chosen because they are spaced about equally over the 22 autosomes and X and Y chromosomes, any unknown disease gene can be roughly localized. The power of this technique comes, in part, from the simple fact that a gene and marker that are close together are less likely to be separated by chromosomal crossing over than a gene and marker that are far apart. Once the approximate position of the disease gene within the genome is determined, other methods are used to locate it precisely and then identify it.

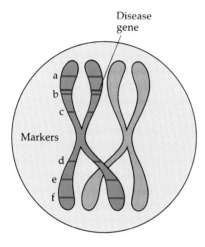

Disease gene

Markers

a
b
c
d
e
f

Crossing over provides information about the physical distance between a marker and a disease gene whose location is being sought. The closer a gene is to a marker, the less likely the two will be separated by crossing over. In this case, the disease gene (red) is closest to marker b. When a parent transmits the disease gene, it is very likely that the polymorphic form of this adjacent marker will also be transmitted to the affected child. This is unlikely to occur with a distant marker like f, which has a much greater chance of being separated from the disease gene by crossing over.

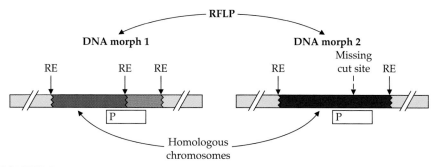

RFLP

DNA morph 1   DNA morph 2

Missing cut site

RE   RE   RE   RE   RE

P   P

Homologous chromosomes

SOUTHERN BLOT

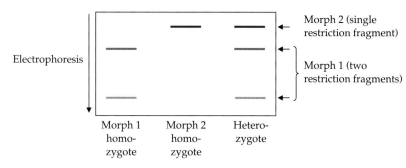

Electrophoresis

Morph 2 (single restriction fragment)

Morph 1 (two restriction fragments)

Morph 1 homo-zygote   Morph 2 homo-zygote   Hetero-zygote

LINKAGE TO D/d LOCUS

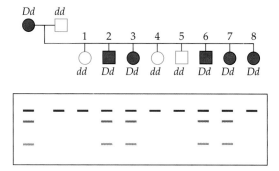

Dd   dd

1   2   3   4   5   6   7   8

dd   Dd   Dd   dd   dd   Dd   Dd   Dd

INFERENCE

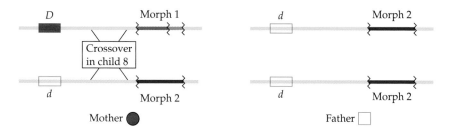

D   Morph 1   d   Morph 2

Crossover in child 8

d   Morph 2   d   Morph 2

Mother ●   Father ☐

The detection and inheritance of a restriction fragment length polymorphism (RFLP). A probe (P) detects two DNA "morphs" when the DNA is cut by a certain restriction enzyme (RE). The pedigree of the dominant disease phenotype suggests linkage of the D/d locus (where D is the dominant and d the recessive allele) to the RFLP locus. (In child 8 crossing over has occurred in the chromosome inherited from her mother. This complicates analysis, but also provides a measure of the distance between the D/d locus and the RFLP locus. The smaller the distance, the less likely a break will occur between the two loci during a crossover.) Before one could conclude with reasonable confidence that the segment of DNA targeted by probe P and the segment of DNA containing the D/d locus are in fact fairly close together on a particular chromosome, a larger number of people in the pedigree (in this or other generations) would have to be examined.

How Genes Work   61

In the past few years, techniques even more practical than Southern blots have been developed to detect DNA polymorphisms that can be used to devise markers. The most popular makes use of an enzyme called *Taq* polymerase (from the bacterium *Thermus aquaticus,* an organism that lives and thrives in the near-boiling temperature found in hot springs). This technique, called the polymerase chain reaction (PCR), can be used to copy specific regions of human DNA that have been found to be polymorphic. In this case the polymorphism being evaluated is not susceptibility to cleavage by a restriction enzyme but, instead, innocuous additions or deletions of short runs of nucleotides.

The original target material is a double-stranded DNA molecule, which is separated into single-stranded templates by heating. Two short sequences of synthetic DNA (called primers), which are complementary to sequences on either side of the polymorphic region in the target DNA, are added to the mixture. The primers will hybridize with these sequences, and *Taq* polymerase will synthesize new complementary DNA strands, beginning from the primer binding sites. From the original single DNA molecule two molecules will be formed, both containing the polymorphic sequences. This replication cycle can be repeated again and again by reheating the mixture to separate the new double-stranded molecules into templates and adding new primers. Because heat-stable *Taq* polymerase (unlike human DNA polymerase) is not damaged by the high temperatures required, it needs to be added only once, at the start of the first reaction; it will remain active from one reaction cycle to the next.

The short DNA segments produced by PCR can then be analyzed by means of gel electrophoresis. In this case, the sample material, which is both unique and very abundant, can be directly visualized by appropriate techniques, and thus a radioactive probe is unnecessary. The type of polymorphism actually detected is a variation in the number of repeats of a particular sequence of nucleotides (e.g., CACA in one form, and CACACACACACACA in another form) in the space between the primers. The number of repetitions determines the length of the PCR products that can be resolved by gel electrophoresis. Like RFLPs, such sequence variations have no harmful effects and are inherited, along with other genes, including disease genes, with which they might share a particular chromosomal region. Since the chromosomal region that binds the particular PCR primers is known, this polymorphism can be used, like RFLPs, to link a region of the genome with a disease.

Because of the potential power of PCR-based analysis, considerable effort, based on this procedure, is being devoted to cataloging polymorphisms throughout the human genome to aid in identifying genes that cause hereditary diseases. This is one goal of an ongoing international effort (which includes the U.S. Human Genome Project) on the part of a large network of cooperating scientists, who hope ultimately to identify, localize, and determine the sequences of all our genes. Their work has already helped isolate and determine the biological function of the genes responsible for such conditions as muscular dystrophy and cystic fibrosis. Attempts to identify genes implicated in major psychiatric disorders, such as manic-depressive illness and schizophrenia, are becoming realistic because of this ambitious program.

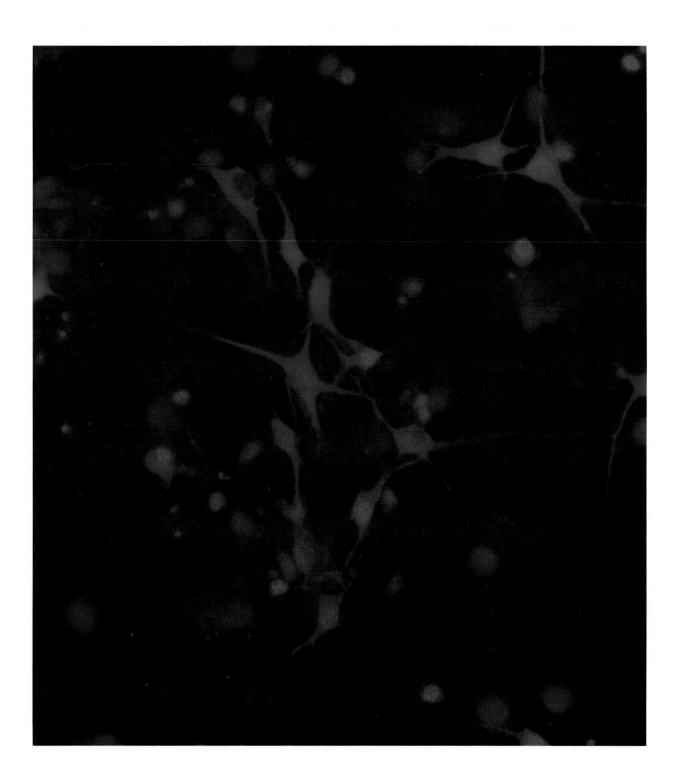

4

NEURONS, CIRCUITS, AND NEUROTRANSMISSION

Thus far, we have considered the genes and proteins that ultimately make brain function possible. But the brain is not simply a random collection of molecules. Instead, it is a highly organized system made up of about 100 billion neurons, a specialized class of cells anatomically and chemically designed for intercellular signaling. The regulated transmission of chemical and electrical signals through circuits formed by chains of neurons is at the basis of all behavior. Consequently, to appreciate current developments in psychiatry, it is necessary to have a basic understanding of the structural and molecular properties that make such intercellular communication possible. The purpose of this chapter is to describe the structure of neurons and the general mechanisms they employ to conduct and transmit signals. Additional aspects of neurotransmission will be considered in subsequent chapters, when the effects of drugs are discussed.

OPPOSITE: Neurons from rat spinal cord growing in a tissue culture dish express an innate property: the ability to extend axons and dendrites to contact other neurons.

Neuronal Structure

Neurons have the same basic structural elements as all other cells in higher organisms. They are surrounded by a plasma membrane composed of lipid and protein, which separates them from their environment, and are filled with an aqueous solution called the cytoplasm, which contains an assortment of soluble enzymes and regulatory proteins. In the cytoplasm are internal structures called organelles, which function as isolated compartments that perform specialized functions. For example, mitochondria provide chemical energy for these very active cells.

Many of the elements involved in the transcription of genetic information are segregated in an organelle called the nucleus. The nucleus houses the chromosomes and is the site of transcription; it also manufactures the ribosomes, structures that assist in protein synthesis, which occurs in the cytoplasm. Folding and certain modifications of new proteins are largely accomplished in two membrane-bound cytoplasmic compartments, the endoplasmic reticulum and the Golgi apparatus. Membranes from these two organelles bud off to form spherical vesicles that are used to build the plasma membrane, which not only forms the neuron's exterior boundary but is also the site where signals are sent and received.

Embedded in the cytoplasm is a constantly changing structure called the cytoskeleton, which is composed of several fibrous structural proteins. These structural proteins are designed to polymerize reversibly into long strands that impart rigidity or flexibility to different parts of the cell, resulting in specific neuronal shapes. They also influence the movements of

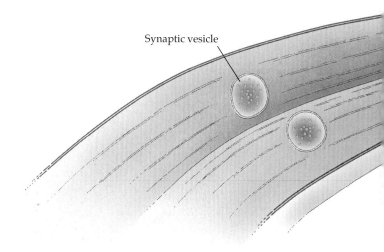

Synaptic vesicle

Facing page: The interior of the cell body of a neuron.

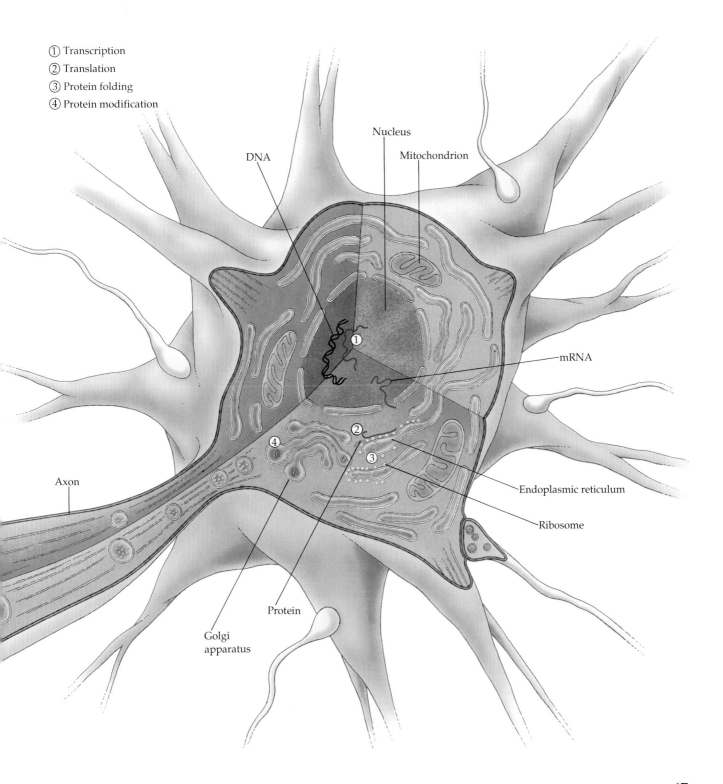

① Transcription
② Translation
③ Protein folding
④ Protein modification

DNA

Nucleus

Mitochondrion

mRNA

Endoplasmic reticulum

Ribosome

Protein

Golgi
apparatus

Axon

67

Dendritic branches receive signals that may be conducted along axon branches and transmitted to other neurons at synaptic terminals. Arrows show the direction of signal flow.

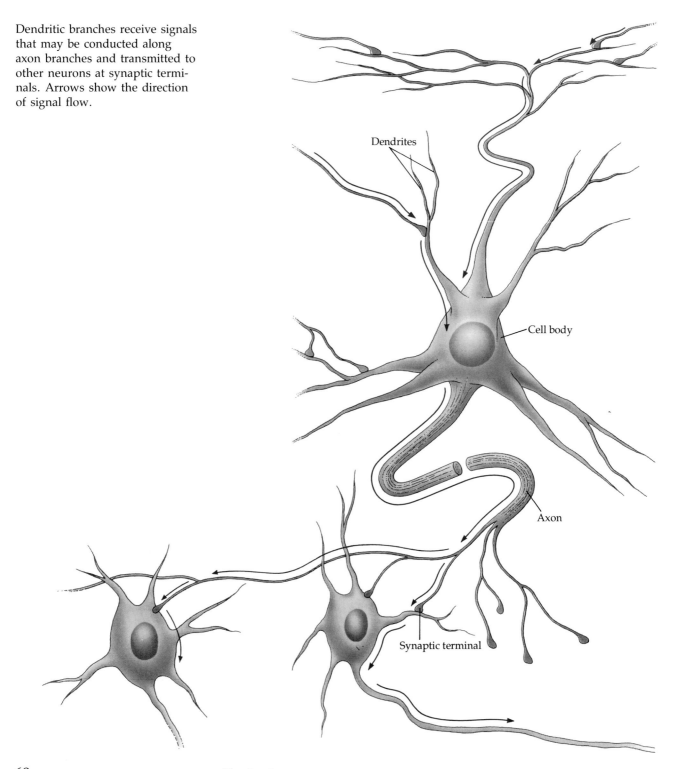

Dendrites

Cell body

Axon

Synaptic terminal

Chapter 4

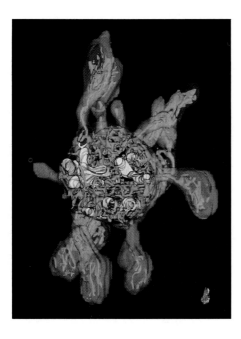

A computer-generated reconstruction of a cross section of a dendrite of a neuron from the brain. Numerous dendritic spines protrude from the dendritic shaft. In this image, plasma membrane is colored gray, endoplasmic reticulum, blue, and mitochondria, yellow. The dendritic spines provide multiple surfaces on which synapses can form.

organelles within neurons, as well as the extension and retraction of cellular projections from the central region, called the cell body.

It is these thin, elongated, and highly branched projections, called dendrites and axons (first examined in great detail by the Spanish neuroanatomist Santiago Ramón y Cajal), that distinguish the anatomy of neurons from that of other cells. Dendrites and axons make possible the extensive interneuronal contacts through which neurons communicate. Dendrites are designed to receive signals from other neurons, especially at small protrusions called spines, and conduct them to the neuron's cell body. The axon is designed to conduct signals away from the cell body along its branches. At the tips of the branches is a further arborization of small protrusions called synaptic terminals, which transmit signals to the dendrites or cell bodies of other neurons. Some neurons contain thousands of synaptic terminals and dendritic spines, making possible extensive contact with many partners.

Signaling occurs at specialized contact sites called synapses, where a synaptic terminal arising from the axon of one neuron (the presynaptic cell) becomes associated with a patch of surface membrane on a dendrite or the cell body of another neuron (the postsynaptic cell). The two components of the synapse are separated by a very narrow space called the synaptic cleft.

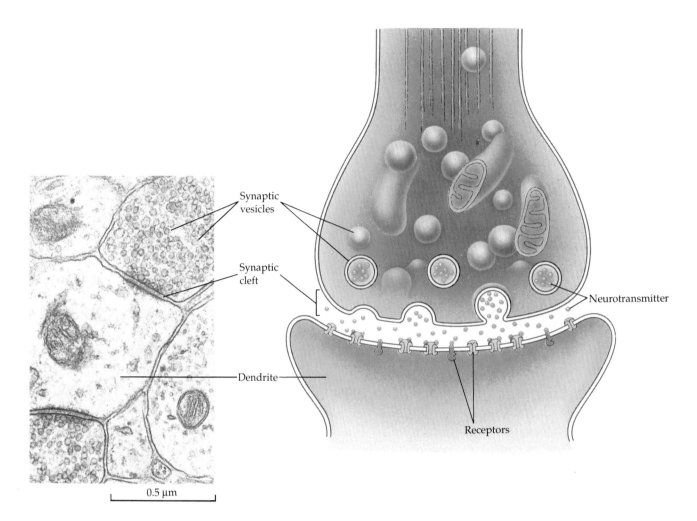

Synaptic vesicles

Synaptic cleft

Dendrite

Neurotransmitter

Receptors

0.5 µm

An electron micrograph and a schematic drawing of synapses. In the drawing, the synaptic terminal is shown activated. Synaptic vesicles are fusing with the presynaptic membrane and releasing a neurotransmitter that binds to receptors on the postsynaptic membrane.

Signals are transmitted across the cleft from the synaptic terminals in the form of chemicals called neurotransmitters, which are stored in membrane-bound vesicles known as synaptic vesicles.

Activation of a synaptic terminal causes the membrane surrounding some of the synaptic vesicles to fuse with the presynaptic plasma membrane. This fusion releases thousands of neurotransmitter molecules, which traverse the synaptic cleft in a fraction of a millisecond and bind to and alter the conformation of specialized proteins embedded in the postsynaptic membrane. When these proteins, called receptors, are activated by a neurotransmitter, certain chemical and electrical properties of the postsynaptic neuron are altered. This is the essential mechanism of cell-to-cell signaling.

Cajal and the Neuron Doctrine

A central concept in this chapter is that the nervous system functions by the interaction of neurons, which communicate with each other via long cellular extensions called axons and dendrites. This essential fact was established by Santiago Ramón y Cajal (1852–1934), a Spanish physician who became the world's leading neuroanatomist.

Cajal's early aptitudes were in painting rather than science. But, having become a physician to please his father, his artistic talents proved invaluable in portraying neurons and their interactions, to the study of which he devoted his life.

At the time Cajal began his microscopic studies, it was generally believed that neurons were fused with their neighbors, forming a continuous network, or reticulum, without the gaps that we now know as synaptic clefts. By applying new staining techniques recently introduced by the Italian neuroanatomist Camillo Golgi, Cajal was able, beginning in 1888, to accumulate evidence that established the physical separation of individual neurons at gaps. This so-called neuron doctrine refuted the then prevalent reticular doctrine, which Golgi himself continued to support as late as 1906, when Cajal and he shared a Nobel prize for their work on the structure of the nervous system.

Cajal's career has many similarities with that of his contemporary, Sigmund Freud. After studying medicine each man became interested in the microscopic anatomy of the nervous system as well as in the use of new stains to reveal

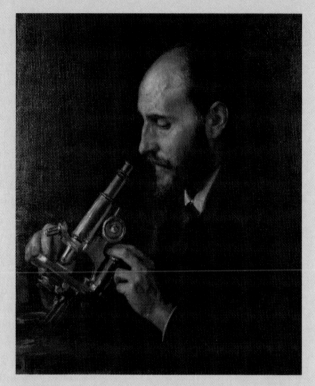

Santiago Ramón y Cajal.

neuronal structure. In fact, in the 1880s one of Freud's aims was the development of a gold-based stain for that purpose—a feat left to Cajal to accomplish many years later. Both also sought to explain the workings of the mind in the language of neurons, a goal that still remains to be achieved.

Neuronal Circuits

Neurons come in many shapes and sizes, and this variability makes possible numerous patterns of interaction. Some neurons have a large number of long dendrites, whereas others have a modest dendritic tree. Some have axons that are more than a meter long, allowing direct communication with distant parts of the nervous system, whereas others have short axons, which are designed to transmit signals to their immediate neighbors. In some cases, extensive axonal branching allows simultaneous transmission to many distant neurons. The basic shapes and branching patterns of neurons and the selection of the partners with which they form synapses are largely determined by the genes that control nervous system structure. The resultant neuronal circuits are the anatomical foundation of behavior.

A very simple example of a behavior controlled by a neuronal circuit is the knee-jerk reflex, which is generally tested in routine physical examinations. This simple reflex involves two principal types of neurons: sensory and motor. The sensory neurons are stimulated by stretching the tendon attached to the kneecap, and they then transmit a signal to the spinal cord. There, the sensory neurons form synapses with the motor neurons controlling the muscles that move the knee. However, even this simple reflex is under the control of other neurons, whose function is to coordinate leg movements during walking. The controlling neurons also make synapses with the motor neurons and may produce complex effects. Some controlling neurons have an excitatory effect, increasing the sensitivity of the motor neurons to sensory stimulation, whereas others have an inhibitory effect, decreasing sensitivity. In fact, one of the reasons for testing the knee-jerk reflex is to determine the activity of a population of controlling neurons that come from the brain and thereby to infer the state of health of the region of the brain in which these neurons reside.

Some neurons participate in much more elaborate circuits. Many involve long chains of neurons, often with divergent and convergent elements. Divergence of axonal branches from a neuron to many synaptic partners coordinates the activity of the postsynaptic cells; convergence of branches from many neurons onto a single postsynaptic cell allows them to cooperate in controlling the flow of activity through this hub. Many circuits also have feedback loops in which a receiving neuron sends axonal branches back to make synapses with the signaling neuron. Given the large numbers of neurons and their elaborate network of contacts, it is not surprising that very complicated behavior results from their interactions.

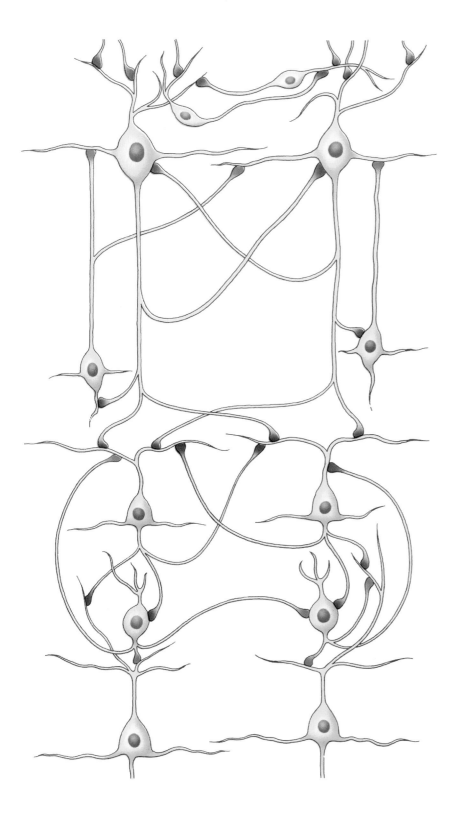

Elements in part of a hypothetical circuit designed to illustrate the main types of neuronal interactions, including convergence and divergence of inputs and feedback. Red shading indicates that a synaptic terminal excites the postsynaptic neuron; blue shading indicates that it inhibits. In reality neurons may receive and send signals from thousands of synaptic terminals. Simultaneous firing of a large number of excitatory synaptic terminals may be needed to excite a postsynaptic neuron sufficiently to propagate a signal (an action potential) along its axon, thereby triggering neurotransmitter release at its own terminals.

Electrical Signaling

The signals transmitted along neuronal circuits are conducted by the movement of charged atoms, called ions, across the plasma membrane, a process that permits transmission at a fairly rapid rate. The process is so efficient (for a biological system) that certain axons can conduct signals at a rate of 100 meters a second. The rates of signal transmission within neurons and the inherent delays involved in chemical signaling across synapses (usually on the order of one millisecond) define the rates at which we can process information and respond to our environment.

Signaling within and between neurons is made possible by the existence of a difference in charge across the plasma membrane of resting nerve cells. This difference, known as the membrane potential, is controlled by a number of regulatory proteins embedded in the membrane that can influence it rapidly and reversibly. To understand how neurons conduct signals, it is necessary to have some appreciation of the general structure of the neuronal plasma membrane and some of its critical constituents.

Like the plasma membranes of all other cells, the neuronal plasma membrane is made up of lipid and protein molecules. The lipid molecules are arranged in a continuous double layer that bars the passage of most substances between the inside and the outside of the cell. Embedded within the lipid bilayer, or closely associated with it, are a number of proteins that control the cell's interaction with its environment. The proteins of major concern for the present discussion are those that are involved in

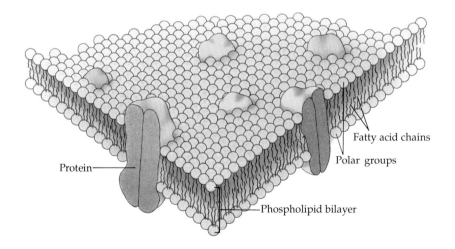

Proteins embedded in the plasma membrane of a neuron. By interacting with the exterior surface of membrane proteins, molecules such as neurotransmitters send signals to the interior of a neuron.

Fatty acid chains
Polar groups
Protein
Phospholipid bilayer

maintaining the neuronal membrane potential and those that regulate its transient changes during neuronal signaling.

Establishment and control of an electrical potential across neuronal membranes is a complex process that will be considered here only in simplified form. When a salt, such as sodium chloride, is dissolved, positively and negatively charged ions are generated. The fluid both inside and outside neurons is rich in these particles. The major positively charged ions, or cations, are sodium (Na^+) and potassium (K^+); the principal negatively charged ion, or anion, is chloride (Cl^-). Neither anions nor cations can pass freely through the lipid bilayer that surrounds the neuron. They can, however, traverse it either passively, through gated channels formed by certain proteins that span the membrane, or actively, via pumps made by other proteins. The channel and pump proteins are generally ion-specific, permitting only ions of a certain size and charge to pass.

The function of the pump proteins is to maintain different concentrations of ions on the intracellular and extracellular sides of a resting neuron's plasma membrane. They and other factors lead to a net negative charge in the neuron's interior as well as to a marked preponderance of K^+ inside the cell and Na^+ outside. The differences in the concentration of particular ions on either side of the membrane, called a concentration gradient, can be reduced by opening channels that permit their passage, since ions will flow from areas of higher concentration to areas of lower concentration to establish equilibrium. Since these differences in charge and ion concentration are separated only by the thickness of the plasma membrane (a very short distance), selective opening of gated ion channels can lead to rapid changes in membrane potential.

The so-called gate in these channels is actually a particular configuration of the allosteric proteins of which it is made. If the configuration is changed, the gate may open, allowing a particular ion to pass. The key needed to open the gate is frequently a neurotransmitter, in which case the channel is called a neurotransmitter-gated ion channel. For example, one neurotransmitter-gated ion channel is formed by a cluster of five protein molecules, several of which bind a neurotransmitter called acetylcholine. Binding of acetylcholine stabilizes the protein cluster in a configuration that opens the channel and permits the passage of Na^+ across the membrane; hence, this channel functions as an acetylcholine-gated Na^+ channel. Since the concentration of Na^+ is much greater outside the cell, Na^+ moves into the cell interior when the channel opens, reducing the net negative charge on the intracellular side of the plasma membrane. The electrical potential across the membrane is thus reduced; that is, the membrane is depolarized.

Activation of a ligand-gated ion channel, in this case the acetylcholine receptor. Binding of acetylcholine to specialized binding sites changes the shape of the receptor protein. As a result, the channel is opened, allowing Na$^+$ to flow through from a region of high concentration outside the cell to a region of low concentration within. This movement of Na$^+$ depolarizes the plasma membrane.

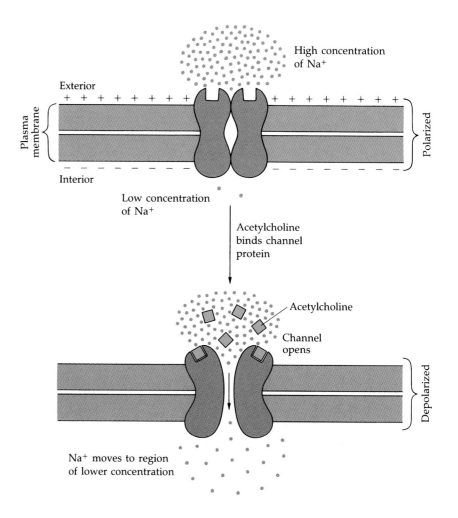

If sufficient acetylcholine-gated channels are opened concomitantly, the plasma membrane of the postsynaptic cell will depolarize enough to trigger a second event along the membrane, namely the transient opening of voltage-gated Na$^+$ channels. The configuration of the proteins that make up this second type of channel are controlled not by the binding of a neurotransmitter but rather by changes in membrane potential. To open them it is necessary to achieve significant depolarization, which may require repeated firing of multiple synapses in the vicinity. This requirement means that a faint signal is ignored; only a concerted call to action excites the postsynaptic neuron.

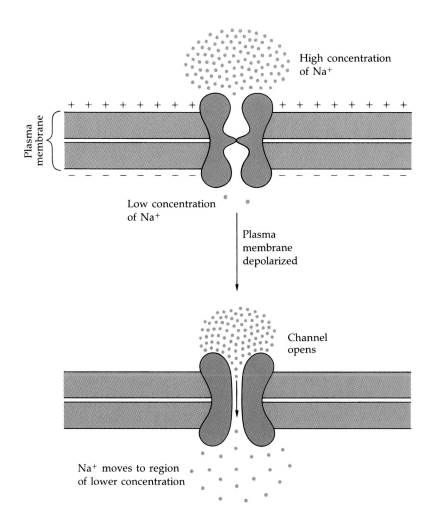

High concentration of Na$^+$

Plasma membrane

+ + + + + + + + + + + + + + + +

Low concentration of Na$^+$

Plasma membrane depolarized

Channel opens

Na$^+$ moves to region of lower concentration

Activation of a voltage-gated ion channel. Normally this protein is surrounded by polarized membrane and its channel gate is closed. However, when the surrounding membrane is depolarized, the channel gate opens, allowing a particular ion (in this case Na$^+$) to flow through. The resulting depolarization may spread to other voltage-gated ion channels in the adjacent membrane.

The opening of the voltage-gated Na$^+$ channels in a section of the postsynaptic membrane sets in motion a chain reaction. This reaction is an all-or-none event. Without sufficient depolarization, it does not take place; but when it is triggered, it is followed by firing in full force, because the entry of sufficient Na$^+$ through a small region of the postsynaptic membrane opens still more voltage-gated Na$^+$ channels, allowing the entry of still more Na$^+$, and causing further depolarization. As a result, a wave of depolarization is transmitted along the plasma membrane of the neuron and down the axon. The self-propagating electrical depolarization along the axon membrane, called an action potential, is responsible for rapidly conducting an electrical signal to the synaptic terminals. The excited neuron now becomes a presynaptic cell, releasing neurotransmitter onto the next neuron in the circuit.

Release of neurotransmitter at synaptic terminals is controlled by another set of voltage-gated ion channels, in this case selective for calcium (Ca^{2+}) ions. When the depolarization conducted by an action potential reaches a synaptic terminal, it transiently opens voltage-gated Ca^{2+} channels concentrated in its surrounding plasma membrane. As with Na^+ channels, the opening of voltage-gated Ca^{2+} channels allows movement of ions from the region of high concentration to the region of low concentration. The relevant moiety is free Ca^{2+} rather than Ca^{2+} that has been sequestered by binding to proteins. The extracellular concentration of free Ca^{2+} is normally about 1000 times higher than its intracellular concentration. This asymmetry is maintained by mechanisms in the interior of the cell that remove free Ca^{2+} from the cytoplasm. One such mechanism involves pumping Ca^{2+} into membrane-bound vesicles, where it is stored until needed.

When the action potential arrives at the synaptic terminal, the voltage-gated Ca^{2+} channels open and free Ca^{2+} rushes in. The resulting increase in free Ca^{2+} in the cytoplasm of the synaptic terminal causes some of its synaptic vesicles to fuse with the plasma membrane and release their highly concentrated stores of neurotransmitter (amounting to thousands of molecules per vesicle). Because only a fraction of the synaptic vesicles in a terminal are emptied with each activation, the synapse can be activated repeatedly. To preclude exhaustion, the vesicles and their contents are also gradually regenerated. However, exhaustion can occur in some circumstances, such as the administration of certain drugs.

Once neurotransmitter molecules are released, they diffuse across the narrow synaptic cleft and bind to receptors on the plasma membrane of the postsynaptic cell. If these receptors are neurotransmitter-gated ion channels, a change in the electrical potential of the postsynaptic membrane results. If sufficient depolarization is produced by the concerted release of neurotransmitter by multiple synapses, the postsynaptic neuron may reach a threshold level of excitation, and propagate an action potential to the next synapse in the chain.

To complicate matters, not all neurotransmitters have an excitatory effect on the postsynaptic membrane. Some neurotransmitter-gated ion channels are selectively permeable to ions that increase the membrane potential rather than reduce it. For example, the neurotransmitter gamma-aminobutyric acid (GABA) opens a gated channel that admits an anion, Cl^-, rather than a cation. Since the extracellular concentration of Cl^- is

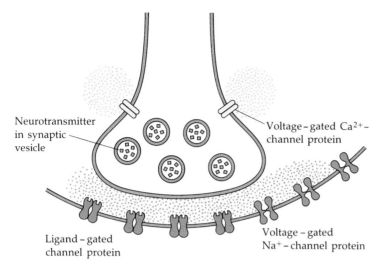

Neurotransmitter in synaptic vesicle

Voltage-gated Ca^{2+}-channel protein

Ligand-gated channel protein

Voltage-gated Na^+-channel protein

Participation of three types of gated ion channels in synaptic transmission. When the synaptic terminal is in the resting state, all channels are closed. With the arrival of an action potential (a wave of depolarization that spreads down the axon membrane), voltage-gated Ca^{2+} channels in the synaptic terminal membrane open, and Ca^{2+} enters. The Ca^{2+} promotes fusion of synaptic vesicles with the presynaptic membrane and release of neurotransmitter. The neurotransmitter crosses the synaptic cleft and opens specific ligand-gated ion channels, depolarizing the post-synaptic membrane. This in turn activates voltage-gated Na^+ channels in the adjacent membrane, spreading the depolarization.

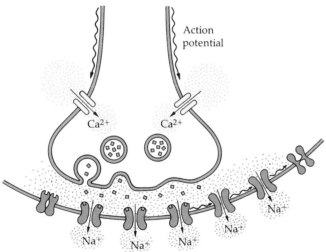

Action potential

Ca^{2+} Ca^{2+}

Na^+ Na^+ Na^+ Na^+ Na^+

higher than its intracellular concentration, opening a Cl^- channel causes Cl^- to enter the neuron. As a result, the interior of the plasma membrane near the open channel becomes even more negative than before, making it less likely that depolarization can occur. Transmitters that open ion channels that increase the membrane potential (i.e., hyperpolarize the membrane) are called inhibitory neurotransmitters. The interplay of inhibitory and excitatory neurotransmitters allows elaborate control of neuronal activity.

The Variety of Neurotransmitters

The complexity of neuronal interactions is greatly increased by the existence of dozens of different neurotransmitters, each with distinctive properties. Several of these signaling molecules are amino acids, including glutamate, the major excitatory neurotransmitter in the human brain, as well as glycine and GABA, the major inhibitory neurotransmitters. Others are monoamine derivatives of amino acids, including dopamine, norepinephrine, and epinephrine (collectively called catecholamines, as they each have a catechol ring), which come from tyrosine; and serotonin (also called 5-hydroxytryptamine or 5-HT), which comes from tryptophan. These monoamines are of great importance in psychiatry, since they have been implicated in mood states, as well as in the experiences of fear and pleasure.

Many other substances released at synapses are peptides that are synthesized as part of precursor proteins and then excised from them by specific proteolytic enzymes that cleave the proteins at particular sites. Like

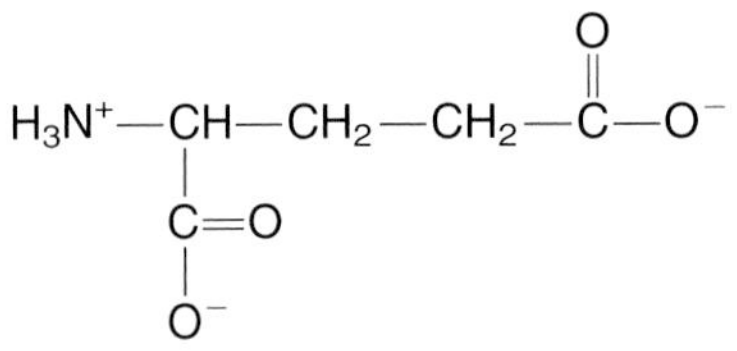

Glutamate

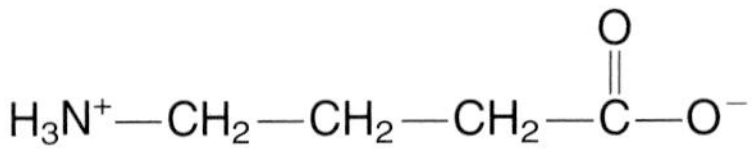

Gamma-aminobutyric acid
(GABA)

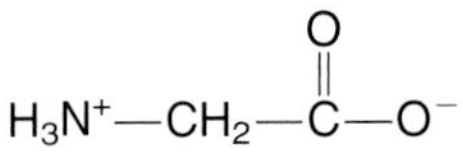

Glycine

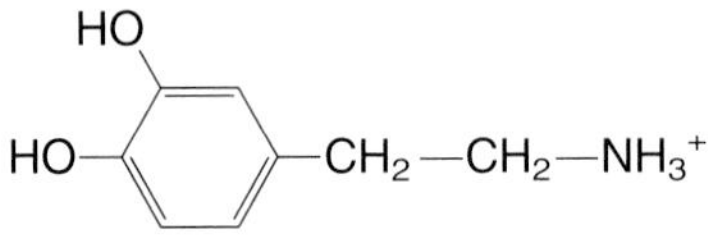

Dopamine

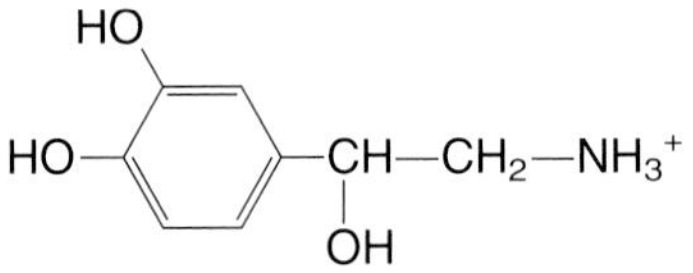

Norepinephrine

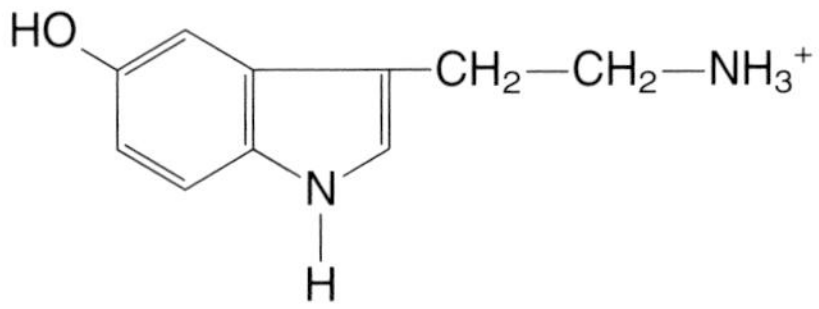

Serotonin
(5-hydroxytryptamine)

many other proteins, these short chains of amino acids (also called neuro-peptides) are encoded by genes that are expressed only in certain cell types. They are often found in neurons along with a nonpeptide neuro-transmitter. In such cases, activation of the neuron may lead to release of both peptide and nonpeptide, permitting complex postsynaptic effects.

In recent years, numerous neuropeptides have been identified. The most widely known are those collectively called endorphins (so designated because their actions are mimicked by morphine and other opiates). The endorphins are actually a family of peptides, including beta-endorphin, met-enkephalin, leu-enkephalin, and others. They are believed to play a role in our perception of pain.

Additional neuropeptides of particular interest are cholecystokinin and corticotropin-releasing factor (CRF). Cholecystokinin, which is found not only in neurons but also in the gastrointestinal tract, plays a role in the feeling of satiety after eating, as well as in the experience of fear. CRF is released by neurons that stimulate the pituitary gland to release ACTH, a peptide that induces secretion of glucocorticoids by the adrenal cortex. As discussed in Chapter 3, the glucocorticoids cause many changes in the body to enhance the response to stressful stimuli. CRF is also found in many other brain regions besides those that stimulate release of ACTH, and may play a role in controlling mood.

A few neurotransmitters are made not from amino acids but from different simple chemicals. For example, acetylcholine is derived from acetate

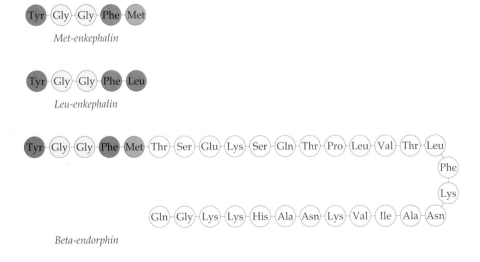

Met-enkephalin

Leu-enkephalin

Beta-endorphin

and choline, the former a biochemical intermediate in general metabolism and the latter a component of certain lipids. Adenosine and adenosine triphosphate, which are derivatives of adenine (one of the four bases in DNA), also may act as neurotransmitters. Some neurons may even release the simple inorganic chemical nitric oxide; however, nitric oxide acts by crossing through neuronal membranes to interact with proteins in the cell interior, rather than by binding to cell surface receptors as a bonafide neurotransmitter would.

Steps in Neurotransmitter Metabolism

One aspect of neurotransmission that deserves further attention is the metabolism of individual neurotransmitters. There are many biochemical steps in the synthesis, storage, release, binding, and inactivation of each of the dozens of different types of neurotransmitters employed in the brain. The overall process is of considerable practical interest, since it is the target of many drugs currently used to treat psychiatric disorders.

Biosynthesis of all the nonpeptide neurotransmitters, such as acetylcholine and dopamine, occurs in synaptic terminals, using enzymes in the cytoplasm. The newly formed neurotransmitters are then packaged in synaptic vesicles to be stored until synaptic terminal activation triggers their release into the synaptic cleft. Since biosynthesis occurs locally, supplies of these neurotransmitters can be rapidly replenished. In contrast, neuropeptides, such as enkephalins, can be made only in the neuronal cell body, where synthesis of all neuronal proteins is segregated. After excision from their large protein precursors, the neuropeptides are transported in a special population of vesicles called dense core vesicles. On arrival at the synaptic terminals, they remain stored in vesicles, like their locally synthesized counterparts, until their release. However, the neuropeptides cannot be resynthesized locally if supplies are depleted; replenishment depends on transport from the cell body and may take many hours.

When neurotransmitters are released, they exert their effects by binding to receptors on the postsynaptic membrane. To terminate this action the neurotransmitter molecules must leave the receptors and be removed from the synaptic cleft. In some cases, removal is achieved by enzymatic degradation of the neurotransmitter. For example, acetylcholine is degraded by the enzyme acetylcholinesterase, which is contained in the membrane of the postsynaptic neuron. If it were not degraded, signaling would continue beyond the appropriate time. Neurotransmitter action may also be terminated by pumping the intact neurotransmitter molecules back into the synaptic terminal that released them. The catecholamines and serotonin are among the molecules whose action is terminated by this mechanism. Reuptake of each of these monoamines is mediated by a specific protein in the presynaptic membrane called a transporter. Individual catecholamines, such as dopamine and norepinephrine, each have their own transporter, as does serotonin. When a monoamine is taken up again by the releasing synaptic terminal, a fraction is repackaged into vesicles and reused; the remainder is degraded by an enzyme called monoamine oxidase, which is contained in the mitochondria of the synaptic terminal. Both the transporters and monoamine oxidase are important targets for drugs used in the management of depression because sustained action of monoamines tends to elevate the mood of these patients.

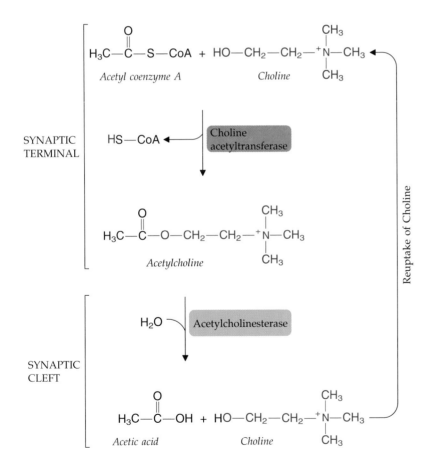

Biosynthesis and degradation of acetylcholine. Biosynthesis occurs in the synaptic terminal and is followed by packaging in synaptic vesicles. When acetylcholine is released into the synaptic cleft it may bind an acetylcholine receptor. Acetylcholine remaining unbound in the synaptic cleft as well as that released from the receptor is degraded by the enzyme acetylcholinesterase, terminating neurotransmission. The choline derived by degradation is transported back into the synaptic terminal and used to make more acetylcholine.

Neuromodulation and Second Messengers

Thus far, we have examined how neurotransmitters act as ligands for gated ion channels, opening a specific channel and changing the membrane potential of the postsynaptic cell. Because this was the first effect of neurotransmitters to be discovered, it is called classical neurotransmission. However, subsequent study revealed that certain neurotransmitters could also have a very different postsynaptic effect by binding to receptors not linked to an ion channel. Since such binding may change the properties of the postsynaptic neuron in ways that modulate the action of channel-linked receptors, the overall process that is set into motion is often called neuromodulation. Many neurotransmitters, such as acetylcholine, may have either effect, triggering classical neurotransmission by binding one type of receptor and neuromodulation by binding another type.

Classical neurotransmission and neuromodulation differ both in their general characteristics and in their specific mechanisms of action. The general characteristics that distinguish them are their latency of onset of action and their duration of action. In classical neurotransmission, the transmitter directly activates a receptor that controls ion flow with an onset latency of less than a millisecond and a duration of less than 100 milliseconds. In neuromodulation the transmitter binds a different class of receptors that set in motion complex intracellular responses whose onset latency may be several seconds and whose duration may be a few minutes or longer. Thus, classical neurotransmission is well suited to generating quick responses and to making neuronal computations that require many steps in rapid succession, whereas neuromodulation is better suited to inducing slower but more durable changes in the state of certain brain functions.

The mechanism of classical neurotransmission has been discussed. That of neuromodulation involves the binding of a neurotransmitter to a class of receptors known as non-channel-linked receptors. Like the neurotransmitter-gated ion channels, these are proteins that are embedded in the postsynaptic membrane; however, rather than forming an ion channel, they function by projecting a specialized tail into the cytoplasm. When a neurotransmitter binds a non-channel-linked receptor, the receptor protein undergoes a conformational change with different functional results than are seen with an activated neurotransmitter-gated ion channel. No transmembrane passageway is opened; rather, the cytoplasmic tail of the receptor protein is altered so that it can now bind a particular member of a class of proteins called G proteins (because their activity is controlled by guanine nucleotides).

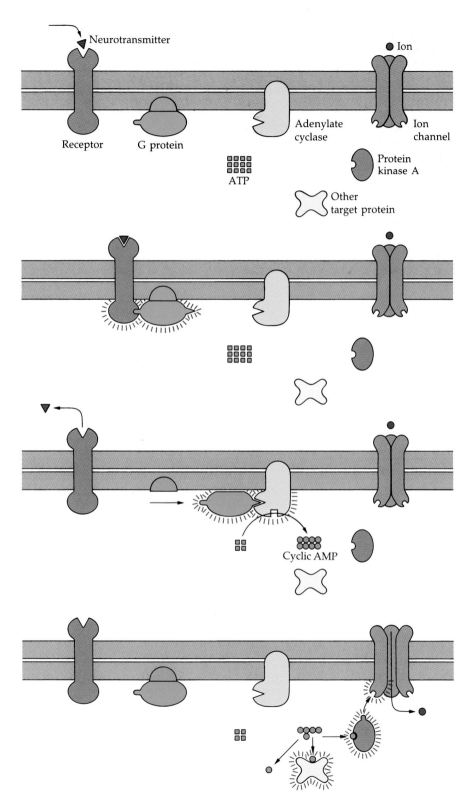

G protein–mediated neuronal signaling. Signaling begins when a neurotransmitter binds to and activates a receptor. The activated receptor can then activate the detachable part of a specific G protein to which it is designed to bind. That specific G protein is also designed to bind to one or more specific effector proteins, such as adenylate cyclase, in this case activating it to manufacture a second messenger, cyclic AMP. Second messenger molecules diffuse through the cell, binding to target proteins, each with different cellular effects. In the case of the cyclic AMP system, one target is protein kinase A, which can in turn phosphorylate an ion channel protein, changing its excitability.

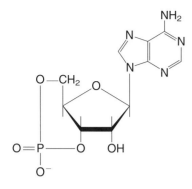

Cyclic AMP

Cyclic AMP, a second messenger. (In the computer-generated model shown above right, and in models in other chapters, the atoms are color coded as follows: carbon (C), gray; hydrogen (H), white; oxygen (O), red; nitrogen (N), blue; phosphorus (P), yellow.)

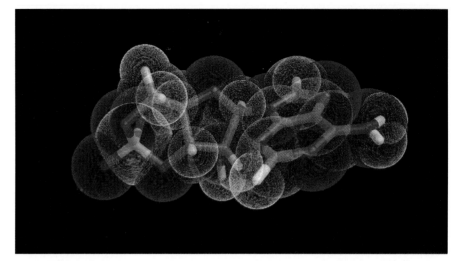

As a result, a detachable component of the G protein is activated, thereby allowing it to interact with and change the function of particular proteins that are its specific targets. The G protein may remain in this activated state for many seconds, mediating changes that last much longer than the 10 to 100 milliseconds a neurotransmitter-gated ion channel remains open. Eventually, the G protein reverts to its resting state, becoming available for another round of activation. However, the intracellular processes it set in motion may last for minutes or even longer.

The most common result of G protein activation is a change in the function of a specialized intracellular enzyme, such as adenylate cyclase. Activated adenylate cyclase synthesizes a great many copies of a small molecule called cyclic AMP, which then spreads through the cytoplasm and may influence the function of many proteins. It may also enter the nucleus and selectively increase expression of certain genes. For this reason, cyclic AMP is called a second messenger; it conveys information to the cell interior from the first messenger, the neurotransmitter.

A major effect of cyclic AMP is to activate an intracellular enzyme called protein kinase A, which incorporates phosphate residues at specific sites in certain proteins, causing conformational changes that have specific physiologic effects. For example, protein kinase A phosphorylates certain neurotransmitter-gated ion channel proteins in neuronal plasma membranes, altering their excitability. This chain of events—activation of a receptor to activation of a G protein to activation of adenylate cyclase to activation of protein kinase A to phosphorylation of the neurotransmitter-gated ion channel—may, therefore, produce a marked change in the excitability of the postsynaptic neuron, making it more or less responsive to other neurotransmitters. This end result may last for minutes or even longer, an essential feature of neuromodulation.

Another intracellular enzyme that may be activated by a G protein is phospholipase C. This enzyme actually generates two second messengers, diacylglycerol (DAG) and inositol trisphosphate (IP_3), by cleaving a plasma membrane phospholipid called PIP_2. DAG then activates the enzyme protein kinase C, which can phosphorylate a number of cellular proteins, including ion channel proteins. IP_3 binds membrane-bound vesicles inside the cell that store Ca^{2+}, thereby releasing this ion into the cytoplasm. Free cytoplasmic Ca^{2+} may directly influence certain ion channels and also activate still other protein kinases that phosphorylate and activate still other ion channels. Therefore, DAG and IP_3 together may modulate the excitability of the postsynaptic membrane.

Activating phospholipase C generates two second messengers, diacylglycerol (DAG) and inositol trisphosphate (IP_3). DAG remains in the membrane, where it activates protein kinase C, whereas IP_3 diffuses through the cytoplasm to exert its effect.

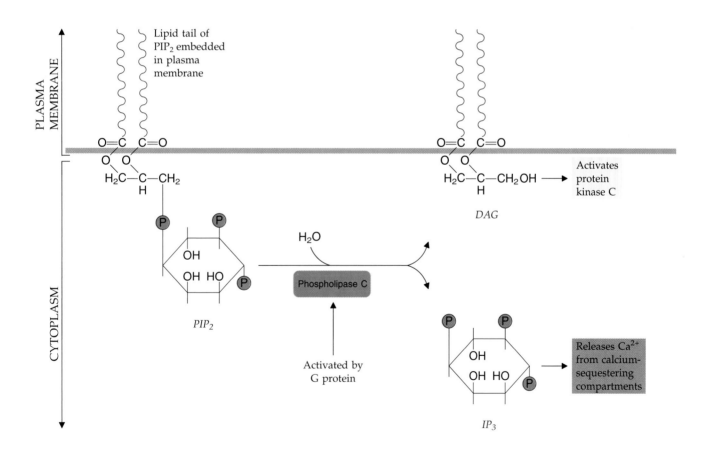

Some Facts about Neurotransmission

1. There are dozens of neurotransmitters.

2. Many synaptic terminals release two neurotransmitters (generally a nonpeptide and a peptide).

3. Each neurotransmitter may combine with more than one type of receptor (generally several, sometimes many more).

4. Some receptors control ion channels, producing transient effects (milliseconds).

5. Some receptors activate specific G proteins, producing more sustained effects (seconds to minutes).

6. There are dozens of different G proteins, each with specific protein targets in the cell (e.g., adenylate cyclase).

7. Many activated G proteins lead to the formation of second messengers (e.g., cyclic AMP) that spread widely.

8. The second messengers may activate certain targets (e.g., protein kinase A) that activate others.

9. Among the targets are ion channels.

10. Second messengers (e.g., cyclic AMP) may diffuse into the nucleus to change expression of certain genes, with long-range effects.

Psychological Effects of Neurotransmitters

It should be clear from this discussion that the large number of different molecules that have been evolved for neurotransmission provides an extremely rich palette with which to generate complex neuronal interactions. This great variety raises the possibility that specific neurotransmitters are deployed in specialized circuits in the brain with particular functions. For example, the monoamine neurotransmitter norepinephrine is highly concentrated in a small number of neurons clustered together in the lower portion of the brain. These neurons project axons and synaptic terminals widely to the brain regions concerned with emotional behavior and information processing. Another monoamine neurotransmitter, dopamine, is mine, is concentrated in other neurons in the lower brain, which also project axons to upper brain regions, but with a different pattern. Together these two neurotransmitters, which activate specific G protein–mediated processes, play complex roles in controlling mood and experiencing pleasure.

One important consequence of the specialization of certain neurotransmitters for specific psychologically identifiable functions is that they offer appealing targets for drugs. It is important to recognize, however, that neuronal signaling has not been designed for the convenience of the psychopharmacologist. Although some transmitters are known to play a dominant role in certain behavioral functions, they are often also deployed in other neuronal circuits, with different behavioral consequences. Furthermore, more than one neurotransmitter may play a critical role in a given behavior. As a result, drugs designed to affect completely different neurotransmitter systems can turn out to influence the same psychological state, such as mood or anxiety. Ways of systematically exploiting the diversity of neuronal chemical signaling systems for specific therapeutic effects are only now beginning to be explored in detail, as we shall consider in the following chapters.

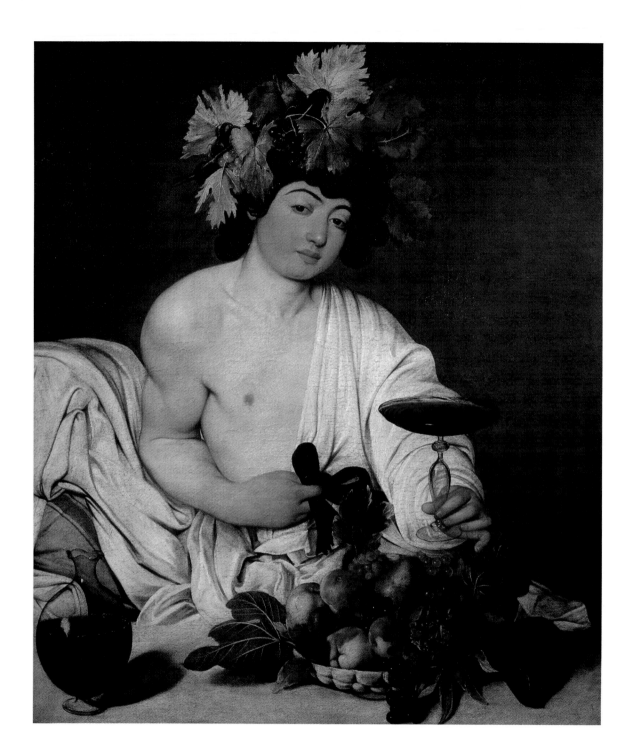

5

DRUGS AND RECEPTORS

Should you have any lingering doubt that the mind is a chemical machine, consider the action of drugs. Since ancient times, people have used chemical agents that altered their behavior. Only in the past few decades, however, have we begun to understand how these drugs affect us and how to develop new ones to treat mental illness. The purpose of this chapter is to provide a broad overview of drugs that affect behavior, in the context of the material already presented. Clinically prescribed and self-administered drugs will be considered together, since they act according to the same principles. The emphasis will be on our growing understanding of how drugs interact with the specific brain proteins involved in neurotransmission. This emphasis will set the stage for subsequent discussion of the use of drugs to treat particular disorders.

—————— OPPOSITE: *Bacchus,* 1589, by Caravaggio. ——————

The Earliest Drugs

The earliest psychoactive drugs were derived from plants. Many of these specialized chemicals are exclusive to a particular plant species and may be present in high concentrations. Some may protect the plants by injuring animals or microorganisms that attack them; but in many cases, the role these chemicals play in the plants that make them is not yet known.

Plant sources of psychoactive drugs have been harvested since ancient times throughout the world. In the Far East, opium was derived from poppies, marijuana from the cannabis plant, and caffeine from tea. In sections of the New World, psilocybin came from mushrooms, mescaline from the peyote cactus, cocaine from the coca plant, and nicotine from tobacco. Alcohol, the most widely distributed psychoactive drug, is unusual in that it is not directly made by plants themselves; instead, it is the product of microbial fermentation of carbohydrates found in all fruits and grains. Our ancestors made use of the drugs in these plants by eating them, drinking their extracts, or volatilizing their active ingredients in smoke. Often they were used in rituals or religious ceremonies to produce altered states of consciousness. In modern times, old drugs have been refined and modified into more potent derivatives, and their use has been secularized.

The remarkable thing about these drugs is that such simple chemicals can produce such profound and reproducible effects on beings as complicated as we are. Small amounts of some of these compounds may change mood, perception, thought processes, and even general behavioral patterns that we think of as part of character or personality. This observation should not be simply taken for granted, since it is not at all self-evident that introduction of a specific molecule into the human brain could have such pervasive and coherent psychological effects. What is particularly extraordinary, as we shall see, is that the actions of psychoactive drugs are not confined to single molecular receptors and neuronal pathways. Because such drugs induce a clearly delineated psychological response, it appears that their minor or extraneous actions can be ignored in favor of their major effect on the overall nervous system.

The use of drugs since ancient times makes the obvious point that their discovery did not require an understanding of the cellular and molecular basis of nervous system function. In ancient cultures, people who became inebriated from drinking fermented grape juice certainly had no knowledge of the biology of the brain, and they often attributed the effects they experienced to spirits or gods. Therefore it should not be surprising that many modern drugs have also been discovered by accident. Given the complexity of the nervous system, it is likely that unexpected actions of drugs will continue to be found and exploited, although a rational psychopharmacology based on predicted actions on specific brain receptors is gradually developing.

The Importance of the Way Drugs Are Taken

Drugs that affect behavior operate by influencing the function of specific proteins in the brain, such as enzymes, receptors, and transporters involved in neurotransmission. To do so, they must reach these target proteins in sufficient amounts to exert a detectable effect. Five steps are involved: (1) ingestion, (2) absorption into the blood, (3) transport to the brain via the circulation, (4) penetration into brain tissue through the membranes that protect it from many chemicals that might disturb it (i.e., the blood–brain barrier), and (5) association with the proteins whose function they control.

Most of an ingested drug dose does not wind up at its target site in the brain. Some of it is not even absorbed, and much remains in the general body fluids, from which it is excreted. These observations suggest that the relatively few molecules that do reach their target sites must bind fairly tenaciously to the proteins that they influence. Indeed, drugs often have a much greater affinity for their target proteins than the native neurotransmitters with which the proteins interact.

Experience with commonly used drugs demonstrates that their behavioral effects are heavily influenced by the way in which they are taken and the rate at which they reach the brain. Cocaine is a good example. When ingested by chewing coca leaves, as was the practice of the Peruvian Incas, cocaine induces a sustained but relatively mild state of increased vigor, which results from the gradual exposure of the brain to cocaine as the drug is slowly absorbed from the intestinal tract. In contrast, when pure cocaine is snorted, absorption is much more rapid, and a wave of euphoria results. Smoking "crack," a volatile form of cocaine, produces an even more rapid onset of action, since the entire dose passes immediately through the absorptive lining of the lung into the blood, and seconds later into the brain.

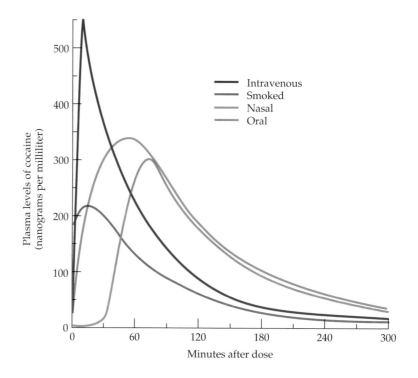

Plasma levels of cocaine after administration by different routes. The oral and nasal doses were each 2 milligrams per kilogram of body weight. The intravenous dose was 0.6 milligrams per kilogram of body weight. The dose smoked was 100 milligrams of cocaine base.

The intense "high" from smoking "crack" is evanescent, the product of a rapid rise in drug blood level followed by a rapid decline.

The circumstances in which drugs are taken also influence their effects. Ambience can be important. For example, the response to a dose of morphine taken postoperatively in the hospital may be very different from the response to the same dose taken as an illicit agent on the street. Both the reason the drug is being used and its anticipated action influence the way it is experienced.

Drug actions may also vary with a person's mental state. Alcohol makes many people feel pleasantly disinhibited but makes others belligerent or depressed. There appear to be more than one reason for such individual differences. In some instances, the person's expectation is important; in others, the response to a drug may reflect biological properties of a particular nervous system.

To date, we have learned a great deal about the diverse behavioral effects of common psychoactive drugs without understanding much about their underlying molecular interactions. This deficiency is now slowly being rectified with the identification of some of the brain proteins whose functions these drugs influence. The greatest progress has been made in identifying the proteins with which drugs interact directly, the drug receptors.

Drug Receptors

Drugs found in plant extracts were useful not only for their behavioral effects but also as the foundation of studies of drug receptors. These studies began in the middle of the nineteenth century with the examination of the influence of drugs on neurons that innervate peripheral organs—such as the heart, muscle, and sweat glands—rather than the more complex neuronal circuits of the brain. In these simple systems, it is possible to examine a single interaction between a neurotransmitter and a postsynaptic cell. The major principle derived from this early work is that certain drugs, called agonists, mimic neurotransmitters, whereas others, called antagonists, block the action of neurotransmitters.

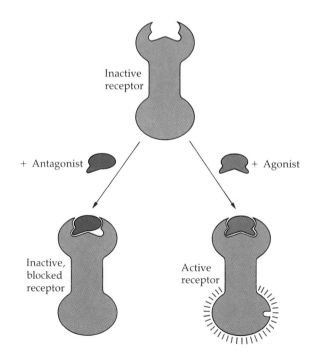

Different effects of binding an agonist or an antagonist. Binding an agonist stabilizes the receptor in an active form (e.g., one that can bind and activate a G protein); binding an antagonist stabilizes the receptor in an inactive form. Since an antagonist occupies the receptor's binding site, it blocks binding of a natural agonist (e.g., a neurotransmitter).

One of the most important drugs used in these seminal studies was muscarine, which was purified from extracts of a poisonous mushroom, *Amanita muscaria*, more than one hundred years ago. Two obvious actions of muscarine are induction of sweating and pupillary constriction, effects that are now known to be due to the drug's mimicking of acetylcholine at receptors in the relevant tissues. Because it produces the same effects as acetylcholine, the natural ligand, muscarine is classified as an agonist.

Unlike agonists, other drugs, called antagonists, do not activate the receptors they bind to. They fit into the receptor protein well enough to block its occupancy by a neurotransmitter, but they do not stabilize the protein in the conformational state necessary to open an ion channel or interact with a G protein; consequently, no direct physiological action is

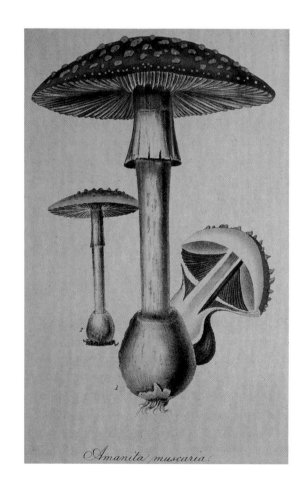

Muscarine

Amanita muscaria.

A computer-generated model of acetylcholine.

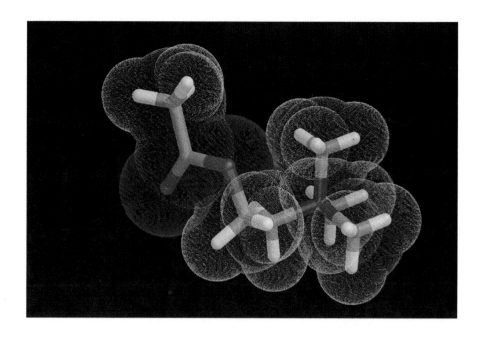

The discovery that muscarine produced physiologic responses that mimicked stimulation of particular nerves and that atropine could block these actions played a major role in the development of early concepts of receptors as materials to which specific chemicals could bind, with different effects. Some time passed before the natural substance that muscarine mimicked was identified as acetylcholine, which was the first neurotransmitter whose chemical structure was definitively established. In a classic Nobel prize–winning (1936) experiment by the German-born pharmacologist Otto Loewi (1873–1961), the neurotransmitter was accumulated in fluid released by electrically stimulating the vagus nerve, which innervates and slows the heart. Since this fluid could itself reduce the heart rate, Loewi directed his efforts at purifying its active ingredient, which was shown to be acetylcholine. Once the chemical structure of acetylcholine was determined, it also became possible to chemically synthesize it in large amounts and to test the effect of the synthetic compound on the heart. The demonstration that synthetic acetylcholine was physiologically indistinguishable from the natural product was the final proof that the real neurotransmitter in the heart fluid had been identified.

Acetylcholine was also shown to be the neurotransmitter that causes contraction of limb muscle (called skeletal muscle); however, this action is observed, although the action of a naturally released agonist is blocked. A classic example of an antagonist is atropine, which was also isolated in the nineteenth century. Atropine blocks the action of acetylcholine (or of muscarine) by associating with receptors to which either of these molecules can bind.

Extracts containing atropine have been used for millennia, for many purposes. The botanical name of the plant from which atropine is derived, *Atropa belladonna*, explicitly identifies two of these. *Belladonna* ("beautiful woman") derives from its cosmetically desirable effect of dilating the pupils of the eyes when taken in small doses. *Atropa* (from Atropos, the name of the Fate who cuts the thread of life) reflects the ancient use of large doses as a poison.

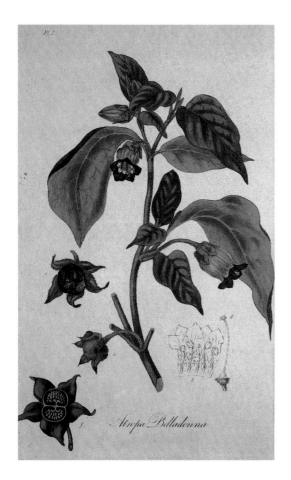

Atropine

neither mimicked by muscarine nor blocked by atropine, indicating that different receptors are involved. In skeletal muscle, two other plant-derived drugs take over the roles of muscarine and atropine: nicotine as an agonist and curare as an antagonist. Nicotine, of course, was derived from tobacco. Curare was obtained from plant samples provided by South American Indians, who, having discovered its paralytic powers, used it to coat the tips of arrows for hunting. We now know that curare causes paralysis by binding to receptors in skeletal muscle in such a way as to prevent acetylcholine from opening the neurotransmitter-gated ion channels that trigger muscle contraction.

Once the two different types of acetylcholine-activated (or cholinergic) receptors had been identified, they were then formally classified on the basis of their responsiveness to drugs, muscarinic cholinergic receptors being responsive to muscarine and nicotinic cholinergic receptors to nicotine. At nicotinic receptors, acetylcholine directly activates a neurotransmitter-gated ion channel and acts as a classical neurotransmitter; at muscarinic receptors, it acts as a neuromodulator through various G protein–mediated processes. Subsequent work has established that there are at least five subtypes of muscarinic receptors and four subtypes of nicotinic receptors, each with a distinct protein structure, different relative affinities for drugs, and different effects on postsynaptic cells.

In addition to agonists and antagonists, there is a third class of drugs, called partial agonists. These drugs bind to a receptor in such a way that it is activated less completely than when bound by its native neurotransmitter. At a quiescent synapse, the net effect of a partial agonist is an increase in postsynaptic activity. At an active synapse, however, in which there is considerable ongoing neurotransmitter release, the effect of a partial agonist is a net reduction in postsynaptic activity, since binding of the native neurotransmitter, which has a greater activating effect, is blocked by the partial agonist. A potentially useful action of a partial agonist would be to keep a postsynaptic neuron in a sustained but moderate state of activity.

Four Drugs That Revolutionized Psychiatry

The growing understanding of the interaction of drugs with neurotransmitters that developed in the first half of the twentieth century had no immediate impact on psychiatry. In fact, the neurons and synapses of interest to pharmacologists were confined to peripheral organs, such as the heart, which had a very simple pattern of innervation. A pharmacology of the brain seemed far too challenging.

There were, of course, drugs available for treatment of general paresis; but these were designed to kill the invading microorganisms rather than influence neurotransmission in the brain. In the absence of other effective treatments, management of the mentally ill during the first half of this century consisted largely of prolonged confinement in asylums. There seemed to be no obvious way of finding drugs that would alleviate such serious symptoms as depression, psychotic agitation, paranoia, and intense anxiety.

The first systematic attempt to develop a drug treatment designed to alter the brain function of patients with serious mental illness was made by Manfred Sakel (1900–1957) at the Psychiatric University Hospital in Vienna, where Freud had studied and where Wagner-Jauregg had developed the malaria treatment for general paresis. In 1933, Sakel introduced a treatment for agitated schizophrenic patients that used insulin, the wonder drug of that period, which had been isolated in 1922 for the treatment of diabetes. Insulin stimulates appetite by lowering blood sugar levels. Sakel and others had made use of this effect by administering small doses of insulin to certain schizophrenic patients who refused to eat. In the course of this work, Sakel noticed that agitated schizophrenic patients were often calmed by this treatment.

This clinical observation encouraged Sakel to experiment with extremely large doses of insulin in the hope of producing a lasting effect. He found that patients who were given large doses of insulin became comatose, sometimes for days, because their blood sugar levels were being kept extremely low. This drastic treatment, called insulin coma therapy, sometimes produced dramatic symptomatic improvement in schizophrenic patients. Although it was impossible to explain how beneficial behavioral effects resulted from starving neurons of sugar, insulin coma therapy became widespread. The attention that this life-threatening and questionably effective treatment received over the subsequent two decades is a measure of the desperate condition of many psychiatric patients at that time.

The situation changed radically in the 1950s with the introduction of four drugs that were both practical and truly effective in mental illness, two for the treatment of schizophrenia and two for the treatment of depression. As with insulin coma therapy, clinical observations provided the initial clues that stimulated the development of these pharmacological treatments. A brief historical account of the discovery of these four drugs will illustrate the circuitous route by which psychopharmacology progressed at that time and by which it sometimes still progresses today.

Reserpine

The two drugs used to treat schizophrenia, reserpine and chlorpromazine, were discovered first. Reserpine was derived from *Rauwolfia serpentina*, a plant that had been used in ancient Hindu medicine to treat both insomnia and insanity. In the 1930s, Indian physicians discovered that it could also be used to treat high blood pressure. This discovery led the Swiss pharmaceutical company Ciba to isolate the active ingredient, reserpine. Working from earlier Indian observations that *Rauwolfia* helped patients with psychotic symptoms, the American psychiatrist Nathan Kline (1916–1984) administered reserpine to patients with schizophrenia. In 1954, he reported that those patients treated with reserpine became calmer, less suspicious, and more cooperative.

One reason Kline's report had a great impact is that it dovetailed with the recent discovery of the monoamines norepinephrine and serotonin in the brain, and with the development of techniques by which these compounds and their metabolites could be measured in biological samples. By means of these techniques, it was rapidly established that reserpine markedly reduced the amounts of both norepinephrine and serotonin in the brain, making these monoamines unavailable for neurotransmission. Shortly thereafter, when dopamine was identified in the brain, it too was shown to be depleted after reserpine treatment. Here, then, was a clinically effective antipsychotic drug whose therapeutic actions could be related to the function of brain monoamines. Unlike insulin coma therapy, therefore, reserpine treatment was not completely mysterious; there were clues to its mechanism of action, and these clues stimulated research on the behavioral functions of the monoamine neurotransmitters.

Chlorpromazine

Implication of a particular monoamine, dopamine, in the schizophrenic process came with another important discovery of the early 1950s, the antipsychotic effect of chlorpromazine. This compound had been synthesized in 1950 by pharmaceutical chemists at Rhône Poulenc Laboratories in France. These chemists had no inkling of the ultimate importance of chlorpromazine in psychiatry: they synthesized it because it resembled known antagonists of histamine, called antihistamines. Any reader who has used antihistamines to relieve symptoms of the common cold knows that such drugs may also be quite sedating.

Both the histamine-blocking and the sedative properties of chlorpromazine were of interest to the French neurosurgeon Henri Laborit. Believing that the antihistamine effect would prevent postoperative respiratory complications and that the sedative effect would relax the patient and facilitate general anesthesia, Laborit gave chlorpromazine to his patients before surgery. He observed that under these circumstances, chlorpromazine exerted a remarkable tranquilizing effect. Excited by these observations, he then suggested that chlorpromazine might also be useful in alleviating the agitation of psychotic patients. In 1952, two French psychiatrists, Jean Delay and Pierre Deniker, followed Laborit's suggestion and found that chlorpromazine was indeed remarkably effective not only in calming schizophrenic patients but also in diminishing their hallucinations and their paranoid thoughts.

Writing in 1970, Deniker recalled the impact of the first clinical trials:

Despite great progress, psychiatric wards of 20 years ago still included agitated patients who did not respond to common therapeutic procedures. Pinel[*] had eliminated chains, but existing treatments could not abolish straitjackets and cells. If we were to recreate the atmosphere of an agitated ward for our students' instruction, they would laugh or become skeptical. . . . Nevertheless, neuroleptic chemotherapy[†] originated in that atmosphere. Logically, a new drug was tried in cases resistant to all existing therapies. We had scarcely treated 10 patients—with all due respect to the fervent adherents of statistics—when our conviction proved correct. It was supported by the sudden, great interest of the nursing personnel, who had always been reserved about innovations.

---

[*]Philippe Pinel (1745–1826), the French psychiatrist who was an early and forceful advocate of the humane treatment of the mentally ill.

[†]A term introduced at that time for antischizophrenic drugs.

The clue that linked chlorpromazine with monoamine neurotransmitters was its alarming side effect: patients treated with large doses of chlorpromazine manifested muscle rigidity reminiscent of Parkinson's disease. At about the same time, it was found that patients with authentic Parkinson's disease had markedly reduced levels of dopamine in the basal ganglia, a region of the brain in which this monoamine is normally concentrated. When taken together, these findings raised the possibility that chlorpromazine might interact with dopamine in the basal ganglia.

It was the Swedish pharmacologist Arvid Carlsson who then related these discoveries to the ongoing work on reserpine. First, he measured brain levels of monoamine neurotransmitters after giving rats either reserpine or chlorpromazine. Reserpine caused a marked decrease in brain monoamines (an effect that was already known), but chlorpromazine, disappointingly, had no effect on brain monoamine levels. Undaunted, Carlsson then measured the breakdown products of monoamines in the urine of rats treated with chlorpromazine and found that the breakdown products of dopamine were markedly increased. This result suggested the novel idea that the brain might be making and releasing more dopamine in chlorpromazine-treated animals in an attempt to compensate for the drug's ability to act as a dopamine antagonist.

After considering all the evidence, Carlsson made the critical inference that the common action of reserpine and chlorpromazine was reduction of dopaminergic neurotransmission. In the case of reserpine, depletion made the drug unavailable for synaptic release; in the case of chlorpromazine, the drug apparently bound to dopamine receptors, blocking dopamine's action as a neurotransmitter. What was particularly exciting about these announcements from the clinic and the laboratory was that not only had two effective drugs for schizophrenia become available, but, for the first time, there was a rational basis for further drug development.

In the mid-1950s, there were two other important accidental findings, both of which proved to be related to neurotransmission by monoamines, and both of which revolutionized the treatment of depression. One was the discovery that iproniazid, a compound originally developed as an antibacterial agent, sometimes improved the mood of people taking it as a treatment for tuberculosis. Since iproniazid was already approved for medical use in humans, this finding and other hints led Nathan Kline, who had already worked with reserpine, to undertake clinical trials of iproniazid's behavioral effects. His studies quickly established that this drug was effective against depression. By 1958 it was being widely used, although its mechanism of action was not yet known.

Iproniazid

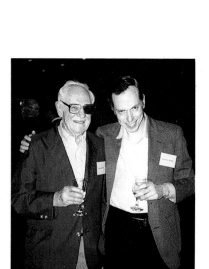

Imipramine

Julius Axelrod *(left)* with his student Solomon Snyder.

Within a few years, the mechanism was suggested by the finding that iproniazid inhibited the activity of monoamine oxidase, an enzyme that participates in the inactivation of norepinephrine, dopamine, and serotonin after their release at synapses. This finding raised the possibility that depression could be overcome by increasing the duration of action of one or more of the monoamine neurotransmitters at synapses, either by retarding their inactivation by monoamine oxidase (as in the case of iproniazid) or by some other means.

Work with still another drug, imipramine, supported the monoamine-prolonging approach to treating depression. Imipramine had originally been synthesized by the Swiss pharmaceutical company Geigy, because its structural similarities to chlorpromazine suggested that it too would be useful in the treatment of schizophrenia. This seemingly rational approach to drug design had an unexpected outcome. Imipramine did not have a favorable effect on schizophrenic symptoms; instead, it was found by the Swiss psychiatrist Roland Kuhn to have significant antidepressant properties.

Kuhn recalls his presentation of the results at the Second International Congress of Psychiatry in Zurich in September 1957:

> We reported the discovery in a paper read to an audience of barely a dozen people. . . . Our paper was received with some interest, but with a great deal of skepticism. This was not surprising in view of the almost completely negative history of the drug treatment of depression up to that time.

Despite the initial reception of Kuhn's work, worldwide studies quickly confirmed the value of imipramine for the treatment of depression. It became the first in a series of variants known as tricyclic antidepressants, which are still widely used to manage this common disorder.

As with the other three drugs mentioned above, imipramine's clinical efficacy was established in the absence of any knowledge of its mechanism of action. Within a few years, however, researchers found that imipramine shared iproniazid's ability to sustain the synaptic actions of amine neurotransmitters; but the two drugs achieved this result in completely different ways. Imipramine's mechanism of action was uncovered by the American biochemist Julius Axelrod, who had already played a major role in elucidating the biosynthesis and degradation of monoamine neurotransmitters, for which he went on to receive the Nobel Prize in 1970.

Axelrod showed that monoamine actions can be terminated not only

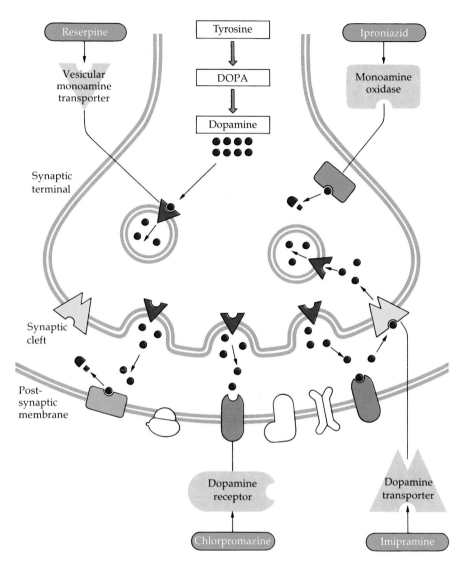

Actions at a dopamine synapse of four drugs that revolutionized psychiatry. Each of these drugs also affects synapses using other neurotransmitters.

by degrading these neurotransmitters with monoamine oxidase but also by transporting them back into the synaptic terminals that released them. In this way, the amines are removed from the synaptic cleft and thus can no longer bind to receptors. Having established the existence of the reuptake process, Axelrod then demonstrated that it was blocked by imipramine

Action of Four Drugs
That Revolutionized Psychiatry

Drug	Molecular Effect	Monoamine Neurotransmission	Clinical Application
Reserpine	Inhibits storage of monoamine neurotransmitters	Decreased	Schizophrenia
Chlorpromazine	Acts as a dopamine receptor antagonist	Decreased	Schizophrenia
Iproniazid	Inhibits monoamine oxidase	Increased	Depression
Imipramine	Inhibits synaptic reuptake of monoamine neurotransmitters	Increased	Depression

and that this blockade prolonged the synaptic effect of all three major monoamine neurotransmitters. Axelrod's work subsequently led to the discovery that there are distinct proteins in presynaptic membranes that selectively transport norepinephrine, dopamine, or serotonin back into synaptic terminals. All three of these transporters are blocked by imipramine; and the serotonin and norepinephrine transporters have become targets for a new generation of antidepressant drugs that act more selectively than imipramine and have fewer side effects.

In little more than a decade, then (from about 1950 to the early 1960s), pharmacological treatment of psychiatric illness was revolutionized in two ways. First, clinically effective drugs for schizophrenia (reserpine and chlorpromazine) and for depression (iproniazid and imipramine) became available. Second, studies of the mechanisms of action of these drugs provided initial clues to the role of monoamine neurotransmitters in both of these abnormal mental states.

Direct Binding Assays of Receptors

Once it was established that clinically useful drugs worked by interacting with brain neurotransmitters and receptors, there was great interest in developing ways of testing other chemical compounds to determine whether they too might have related therapeutic effects. One way of evaluating therapeutic efficacy is to examine the effects of various drugs on specially developed tests of animal behavior; however, animal studies are very time consuming and expensive, and are often difficult to interpret.

A more convenient way is to compare the interaction of a series of drugs with a receptor by means of a procedure known as a direct binding assay. This procedure (depicted on the following page), which was brought into wide use by Solomon Snyder and colleagues at Johns Hopkins University, measures the degree to which a drug binds to receptors that are present in fragments of synaptic membranes. First, the membrane fragments are prepared by chopping up bits of brain. The fragments are then incubated with radioactively labeled neurotransmitters or radioactively labeled drugs, so that they may bind to one (or more) of the different receptors embedded in the membranes. After all of the unbound radioactive ligand is washed away, the amount of the drug or neurotransmitter that remains bound to the receptors is estimated by measuring the radioactivity associated with the membrane fragments.

Data from direct binding assays form the basis for comparative studies of the relative affinity of different drugs for a given receptor. If, for example, a fixed amount of a radioactively labeled ligand is mixed with increasing amounts of a nonradioactive drug and the mixtures are exposed to the synaptic membrane fragments, the amount of nonradioactive drug required to displace the radioactive ligand can be determined. Other nonradioactive drugs can be tested in this way as well, and the results compared. This provides a measure of the relative affinity of each of the drugs for the receptor, which should correlate with their efficacy as pharmacological agents in neuronal systems that use this receptor type.

Although we tend to think of drugs as binding exclusively to a single receptor, the reality is that many drugs can bind to several different receptors, with varying affinity. One important application of direct binding assays is to develop a profile of the relative affinities of a series of drugs for a number of different receptors, which can then be compared with the relative effects of these same drugs on a psychiatric symptom. For example, chlorpromazine, as we have seen, was first developed to bind to hista-

The principle of a direct binding assay. Membranes derived from chopped-up brain tissue are reacted with a radioactive ligand (red dots), in this case dopamine. This ligand binds to the receptors in the membranes but is displaced by nonradioactive ligands, here two drugs (blue or green dots). The relative affinity of different drugs for a receptor can be estimated by the amount of radioactive ligand each displaces.

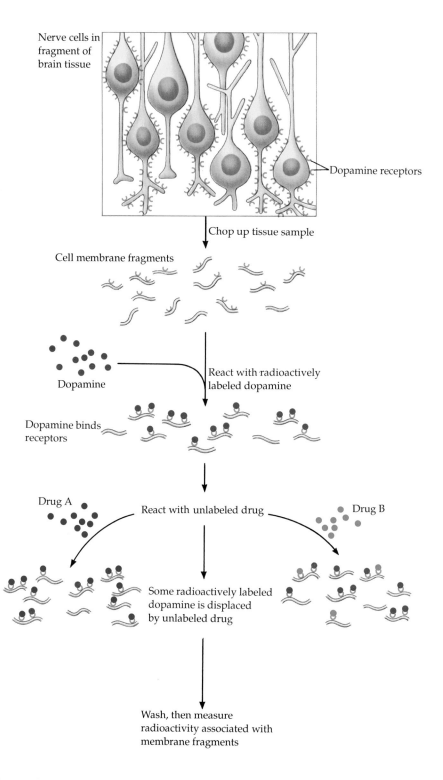

Nerve cells in fragment of brain tissue

Dopamine receptors

Chop up tissue sample

Cell membrane fragments

Dopamine

React with radioactively labeled dopamine

Dopamine binds receptors

Drug A

React with unlabeled drug

Drug B

Some radioactively labeled dopamine is displaced by unlabeled drug

Wash, then measure radioactivity associated with membrane fragments mine receptors but was subsequently found to bind to dopamine receptors. Some compounds related to chlorpromazine share only the first binding property, whereas others share only the second. Only those drugs that bind well to dopamine receptors alleviate psychotic symptoms; those that bind well only to histamine receptors do not. Thus, it is the dopamine receptors rather than the histamine receptors that are the real targets of the antipsychotic effect.

Cloning Receptors

Although binding studies using crude brain membrane preparations have proved useful in characterizing the properties of many drugs, they are of little value in examining scarce brain receptors, because the amount of drug or neurotransmitter these receptors bind may be too small to measure. Furthermore, the binding of a drug to scarce receptors in crude membrane preparations may be obscured if the drug also binds to other receptors that are very abundant. Since scarce receptors may be of vital importance for a particular brain function, there is great interest in obtaining pure samples of these proteins, so that they can be made available in the amounts required for drug binding studies. However, purification of scarce receptor proteins from brain tissue has proved to be very difficult technically.

Fortunately, the problem of obtaining sufficient amounts of scarce receptors was solved by a new approach. Rather than trying to isolate these scarce proteins from the brain, researchers found a way of making them in limitless quantities in the test tube. Since this powerful and elegant approach is so critical for an appreciation of contemporary research in psychopharmacology, I will briefly review its essential features.

As we saw in Chapter 3, for a cell to manufacture proteins (such as receptor proteins), it must contain the mRNAs from which they were translated. In fact, every neuron contains thousands of different mRNAs, with each mRNA controlling the synthesis of a specific cellular protein. If it were possible to isolate the mRNA that encodes a specific receptor protein, it might then be translated into limitless copies of this protein. A series of techniques to achieve this goal have been devised.

Development of these techniques depended on several discoveries. The first was made in 1970 in the course of studies examining how viruses composed of RNA (such as the virus responsible for AIDS) make the DNA needed to replicate themselves. RNA viruses accomplish this task with the help of an enzyme known as reverse transcriptase, so called because it transcribes DNA from RNA, the reverse of the normal flow of genetic information. The product of this reversed transcription is a population of DNAs whose base sequences are complementary to the population of mRNAs in the selected tissue. For this reason, they are called complementary DNAs, or cDNAs. When first copied from mRNAs, they consist of a single complementary strand; but single-stranded cDNA can be used as a template to make double-stranded cDNA.

The next critical advance was a technique that allowed researchers to make multiple copies of each of the cDNAs and to fish out the specific cDNA that encodes the receptor of interest. Although there are now many permutations of this procedure, the pioneering work was done in 1973 by Herbert Boyer at the University of California at San Francisco and Stanley Cohen at Stanford University.

The first step is to splice individual double-stranded cDNAs into small circular pieces of appropriately modified bacterial DNA, called plasmids. Since the small bit of cDNA is being combined with the plasmid's DNA, the product is called recombinant DNA. The resultant plasmids, each incorporating an individual cDNA molecule, can then be introduced into specially prepared bacterial cells. Each bacterium gets one plasmid with a particular cDNA. This mixed population of cDNAs, derived from the original tissue sample and propagated in bacteria, is called a cDNA library.

The next step is to separate each member of the library from all others so that the particular cDNA of interest can be isolated. This is achieved by growing the bacteria on a solid nutrient agar surface at low density, so that each bacterium in the library is separated by a large distance from the others. Since the bacteria stay in place as they grow and divide on the nutrient agar, each bacterium will generate an isolated colony of descendants, called a clone. Each member of the clone contains copies of the plasmid with the particular cDNA contained in the clone's founder.

The challenge, then, is to locate a single clone among the thousands of clones present. Many different techniques have been developed to accomplish this task. Several of these involve expressing the information in the cDNA by transcribing mRNA from it and then translating the mRNA into the receptor protein. For many applications, the entire process is completed in the bacterial clone that contains the cDNA. To study brain receptors, however, it is necessary to transfer the plasmid with the cDNA to cultured human cells, because the human cells insert the receptor protein into their membranes in a manner that facilitates its detection by drug or neurotransmitter binding.

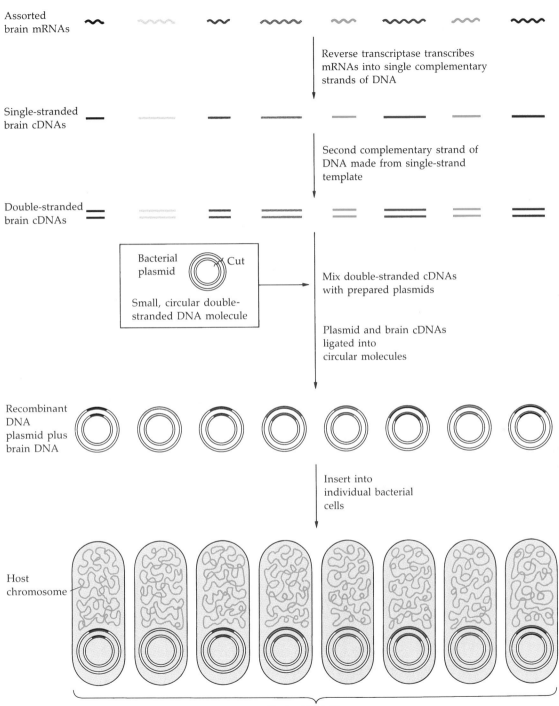

Assorted
brain mRNAs

Reverse transcriptase transcribes
mRNAs into single complementary
strands of DNA

Single-stranded
brain cDNAs

Second complementary strand of
DNA made from single-strand
template

Double-stranded
brain cDNAs

Bacterial
plasmid   Cut

Small, circular double-
stranded DNA molecule

Mix double-stranded cDNAs
with prepared plasmids

Plasmid and brain cDNAs
ligated into
circular molecules

Recombinant
DNA
plasmid plus
brain DNA

Insert into
individual bacterial
cells

Host
chromosome

Brain cDNA library

Since it is impractical to test the thousands of clones in the library one at a time, the search is conducted in steps. First, the library is divided into pools, each of which contains a fraction of the clones, and the pools are screened for the receptor. The pool found to have the desired cDNA is divided into further pools, and screening is repeated. Ultimately, a single clone is obtained that contains only the receptor cDNA. Although this account oversimplifies certain technical issues, it captures the essential power of this technology. Beginning only with the knowledge that a specific drug works on the brain or that a specific neurotransmitter must have a receptor, one can eventually isolate the particular cDNA that encodes the receptor.

Once the clone that contains the cDNA for the receptor has been isolated, the sequence of nucleotides in the cDNA can be determined by means of a well-established simple chemical procedure, and the receptor's precise amino acid sequence can be deciphered. Knowledge of the amino acid sequence is useful for many purposes, including studies of the three-dimensional structure of the receptor. Furthermore, once the pure clone is available, it can be grown in limitless quantities; human cells that express it can be used to study drug-receptor interactions and to evaluate new drugs.

Drug-Induced Brain Changes

Thus far, we have considered drug actions in terms of what happens immediately upon their administration. But drugs, as normally used, do not act only instantaneously: their effects may last for hours or even days. Furthermore, drugs are frequently given in repeated doses, so that they exert their effects over a period of weeks, months, or years. In addition, sustained administration of drugs itself alters the brain in many ways, and such alterations may, in turn, change the drugs' effects.

Brain changes may occur within seconds or minutes of drug administration. For example, repeated stimulation of postsynaptic receptors by an agonist may quickly lead to cellular changes that inactivate the receptors. One such change is phosphorylation of postsynaptic receptors stimulated by second messengers and protein kinases. The phosphorylated receptors may become incapable of another round of activation until the phosphate residues are removed.

A more sustained process, called down-regulation, is brought into play by continued exposure to an agonist. In these circumstances, receptors

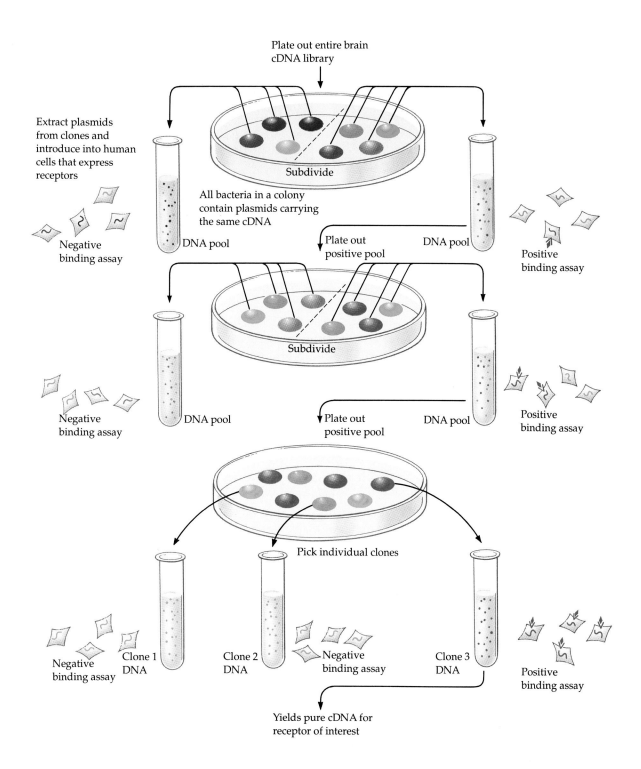

Plate out entire brain cDNA library

Extract plasmids from clones and introduce into human cells that express receptors

Subdivide

All bacteria in a colony contain plasmids carrying the same cDNA

Negative binding assay

DNA pool

DNA pool

Positive binding assay

Plate out positive pool

Subdivide

Negative binding assay

DNA pool

Plate out positive pool

DNA pool

Positive binding assay

Pick individual clones

Negative binding assay

Clone 1 DNA

Clone 2 DNA

Negative binding assay

Clone 3 DNA

Positive binding assay

Yields pure cDNA for receptor of interest

113

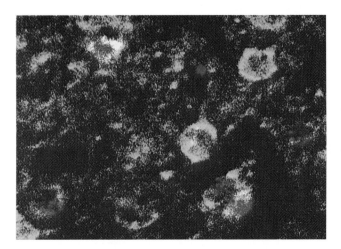 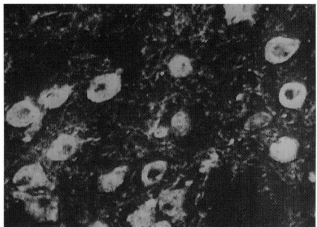

Cocaine causes increased expression of a transcription factor in the nuclei of certain neurons in the basal ganglia of rat brain. A rat was given cocaine, which blocks reuptake of dopamine at synaptic terminals, causing increased activation of postsynaptic dopamine receptors. Two hours later the rat was sacrificed and a portion of the basal ganglia was stained with two antibodies, each of which detects a specific protein. The green antibody detects a protein called DARPP-32 that is present in many neurons that respond to dopamine. The red antibody detects a protein called Fos, a transcription factor that controls the expression of many genes. The intense red staining in the nuclei of some of the neurons in the photo on the left is due to increased expression of Fos after cocaine administration. The photo on the right is from a control rat not treated with cocaine. There is no Fos in any of the nuclei.

begin to be withdrawn from the membrane of the postsynaptic cell, or the rate at which new receptors are inserted slows. The result is a loss in sensitivity to the agonist that may last for hours, until the normal number of receptors is restored. Receptor phosphorylation and removal of receptors from the cell surface are components of a general process called desensitization, in which sensitivity to a drug may be lost even while a dose is still in the body. Antagonists may drive this process in reverse, rendering synapses hypersensitive.

More complex reactions may occur in postsynaptic neurons, especially with repeated drug administration. These reactions, typically set in motion by second messengers (e.g., cyclic AMP), may be due to increased or decreased expression of particular genes in the postsynaptic cells, some of which are quickly activated and therefore are called immediate-early genes. For example, cocaine, which prolongs the action of dopamine at synapses, activates a gene called c-*fos* in the postsynaptic neurons within minutes after the drug is taken. The effect is mediated by increased cyclic AMP in the postsynaptic neuron. The activated c-*fos* gene makes the Fos protein, which is a transcription factor for other neuronal genes. Since the Fos protein carries the neurotransmitter's message beyond that of the second messenger, it is sometimes called a third messenger. It may give rise to a complex series of changes in the protein composition and function of the postsynaptic neuron.

Drugs used in the treatment of mental illness also produce complex changes in the nervous system, and there is reason to believe that in some

Chapter 5

cases, those changes, rather than the drugs' acute actions, are responsible for the therapeutic effects. For example, imipramine immediately blocks synaptic reuptake of monoamines; but it may not exert its antidepressant effect until repeated doses are taken over several weeks. The inference is that it takes that long to produce the chemical changes in the brain that alleviate depression. Some of these changes may actually occur in neurons that are not directly affected by imipramine but become secondarily involved as members of the same neuronal circuits.

In view of the complicated effects of drugs on our brains and our behavior, it is little wonder that progress in identifying new drugs has depended so heavily on accidental discoveries. Nevertheless, the growing understanding of the molecular actions of drugs is becoming increasingly important in the development of new variants as well as new classes of active compounds. This will become apparent as we consider the treatment of psychiatric disorders in greater detail in the chapters that follow.

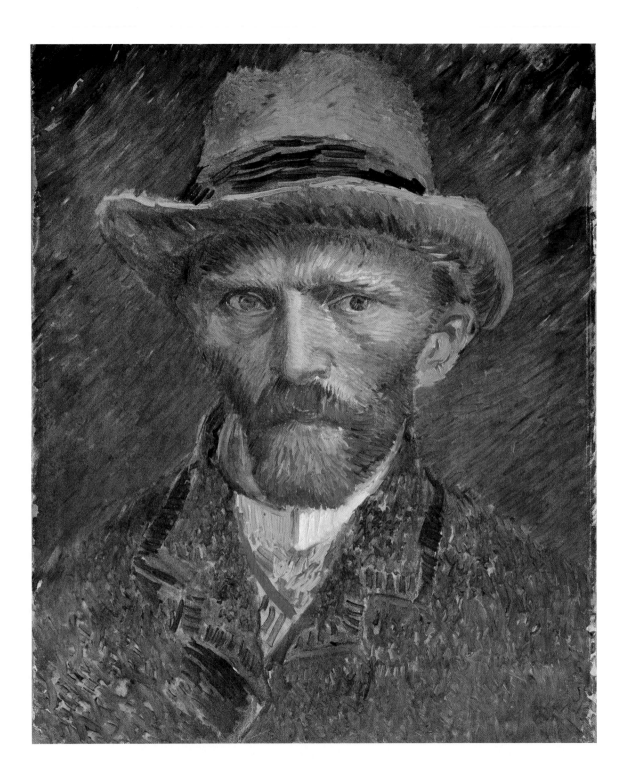

6

MANIA AND DEPRESSION

In the past few chapters, we have presented evidence that individual molecules and the biological mechanisms they control are critical building blocks of behavior. We have also seen how research at the molecular level has made great contributions to psychopharmacology and behavioral genetics. We will spend the remaining chapters examining major psychiatric disorders from precisely this molecular perspective. What light have advances in pharmacology and genetics already shed on the nature of profound mental disturbances such as manic-depressive illness and schizophrenia? How will those advances contribute to future advances in diagnosis and treatment?

Mood disorders are a good starting point for considering the applications of biological research to psychiatry because we have already learned a

OPPOSITE: *Self-Portrait, in Gray Felt Hat* by Vincent van Gogh, who had bipolar disorder that culminated in suicide.

great deal about drugs that influence mood and there is particularly strong evidence for an inherited predisposition to manic-depressive illness. Before we address these topics, let us consider the normal function of moods and the difference between normal fluctuations in mood and a mood disorder.

Evolutionary Value of Moods

All of us are personally familiar with good moods. At times, we are content, optimistic, even expansive; we like to be with people, and they like to be with us. Such states of happiness may be transient conditions for some and virtually perpetual for others.

All of us also know what it means to be sad. In such a state we tend to be suspicious and pessimistic. We think poorly not only of our prospects but also of ourselves. We tend to stay away from people, and they, sensing our discomfort, tend to stay away from us. Even when good things happen, we derive little pleasure from them. Like states of happiness, states of sadness may be either transient or sustained.

All of us also have some knowledge of more extreme moods. We have felt or observed grief at the loss of a loved one; we know about the elation that accompanies some great good fortune. It is also likely that we have encountered someone in a sustained and serious depression or maybe even witnessed an ebullient and irresponsible manic episode.

But rarely, if ever, do we ask ourselves why moods exist in the first place. What is the biological function and the evolutionary advantage of this dimension of our behavior? Might our species not be better off if we took both good and bad in stride, without any change in mood?

There are probably a number of reasons why mood evolved. The most obvious is that mood is part of the mechanism by which our brains register and process rewards and punishments. When we are rewarded for a behavior, we feel good; when we are punished, we feel bad. These sustained feelings, our moods, themselves become rewards we seek or punishments we avoid.

In addition to its role in individual behavior, mood also fosters certain human social patterns that are critical for our survival. Since we are intensely social animals, completely dependent on parents for our early nurturance and on social structure for our defense and prosperity, traits that promote and sustain social bonds have obvious evolutionary value.

The best evidence for mood as a socializing agent is the persistent melancholy caused by separation from a loved one. This reaction has been extensively studied in infants and young children, who, when separated from their mothers, initially express protest but ultimately experience despair. To keep the infant (and herself) from feeling sad, the mother tries to limit separation. In later life, the sadness we feel at separation signals us to avoid this unpleasant feeling and fosters affiliation.

Mood may also be critical for establishing group structure and determining leadership. For instance, we tend to follow the upbeat person and avoid the melancholic. This inclination often proves useful since the confident and energetic leader tends to be full of new ideas and creative solutions. Because such charisma may be critical for the prosperity of groups, elevated mood may have evolved as a way of inducing certain individuals to lead and others to follow.

To serve any of these functions, however, moods are useful only in moderation. When they exceed a certain intensity they become destructive. For example, the bitter, sustained, and deep depressions that some of us experience can only be detrimental to ourselves and others. No obvious redeeming value is offered by depressions to the point of thoughts of worthlessness and suicide, or by manic episodes characterized by frenzied activity and poor judgment. But where is the boundary between normal mood and mental illness?

Distinguishing Normal and Abnormal Moods

In *Billy Budd, Sailor,* the novelist Herman Melville, who himself suffered from recurrent and severe depressive episodes, posed the problem of distinguishing between normal and abnormal moods metaphorically (and with considerable poetic license about the order of colors in the rainbow):

> Who in the rainbow can draw the line where the violet tint ends and the orange tint begins? Distinctly we see the difference of the colors, but where exactly does the one first blendingly enter into the other? So with sanity and insanity.

Despite the blurred borders, mood disorders are usually easy to distinguish from normal mood fluctuations. Consider the personal experience of depression described by the poet Sylvia Plath in *The Bell Jar:*

> I hadn't slept for seven nights. . . .
>
> The reason I hadn't washed my clothes or my hair was because it seemed so silly.
>
> I saw the days of the year stretching ahead like a series of bright, white boxes, and separating one box from another was sleep, like a black shade. Only for me, the long perspective of shades that set off one box from the next had suddenly snapped up, and I could see day after day after day glaring ahead of me like a white, broad, infinitely desolate avenue.
>
> It seemed silly to wash one day when I would only have to wash again the next.
>
> It made me tired just to think of it.
>
> I wanted to do everything once and for all and be through with it.

Consider also the manic behavior of the following patient, described by the American psychiatrist Ronald Fieve in *Moodswing:*

> All by himself, he had been building a magnificent swimming pool for his country home in Virginia, working 18 hours a day at it. He decided to make the pool public and open the concession stand at one end to help defray the mounting costs of the project. When his wife suggested that he might be going overboard, he became furious and threatened to leave her for another woman. Soon afterward, when his wife was out, he took many valuables from the house—his share, he claimed—and sold or pawned them. Complaining that his wife was a stick in the mud, he decided to throw a round-the-clock party, and he invited to the house almost everyone he passed on the street. This psychotic behavior went on for weeks, and during this time he slept only two to four hours a night. He had no time to eat, and he talked continuously, planning grandiose sexual schemes "as soon as someone takes my wife off my hands."

What Plath described are typical accompaniments of severe depression: intractable insomnia, indifference to grooming, the feeling that nothing is worthwhile. Fieve's patient was in the throes of a manic episode: extremely energetic, throwing money around, hypersexual, grandiose.

But do such symptoms constitute an illness? Since Plath killed herself at the age of 31, it is difficult to conclude that what she was feeling was within the normal range of moods. Fieve's patient also was headed for serious difficulties, at least maritally and financially. But at what point do high moods or low moods become symptoms of a disease?

Defining Syndromes and Mental Disorders

When we speak of illness, we generally assume that two things are present: a demonstrable pathology and a detectable cause. For example, general paresis, considered in Chapter 1, is caused by a microorganism that gives rise to gross brain destruction. Likewise, Huntington's disease, considered in Chapter 2, is the result of an abnormal gene that causes certain neurons to degenerate.

With mood disorders (and other psychological disorders we will consider later), the situation is different, since to date we have been unable either to demonstrate obvious brain abnormalities or to establish a definite etiology. The only defining characteristics of mood disorders are patterns of behavior that resemble, but exceed, what normal people display.

In medicine, a pattern of symptoms is called a syndrome. For example, the syndrome called anemia includes pallor, tiredness, and shortness of breath. Any one of these symptoms may be displayed by normal people and need not be a signal of disease. Only the pattern—the syndrome—suggests illness.

Once the syndrome is defined, it becomes the basis for research into the cause. In the case of anemia, such research led to the discovery that certain patients had characteristic abnormalities in either the size or the shape of their red blood cells and that these patients could be classified into separate categories on the basis of these abnormalities. This discovery, in turn, helped distinguish a number of different nutritional diseases (such as iron deficiency anemia) and genetic diseases (such as sickle-cell anemia), each of which produces the syndrome of anemia.

Psychiatry too has its syndromes. In the United States, they are formally defined in the *Diagnostic and Statistical Manual of Mental Disorders*, published and updated by the American Psychiatric Association. The current version, *DSM-III-R* (which will be replaced in 1993 by *DSM-IV*), explicitly discusses the general issue of defining mental disorders as follows:

> Although this manual provides a classification of mental disorders, no definition adequately specifies precise boundaries for the con-

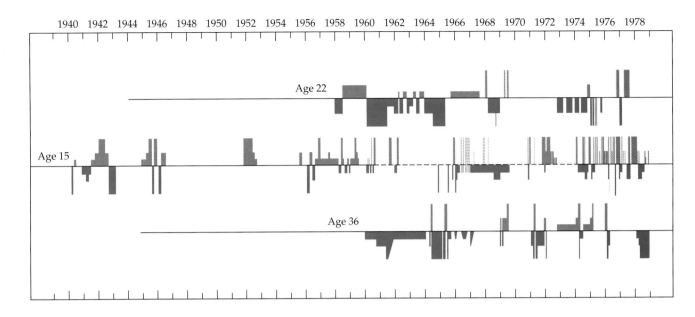

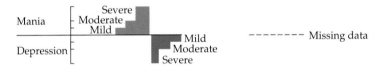

Manic and depressive episodes in three patients with bipolar disorder.

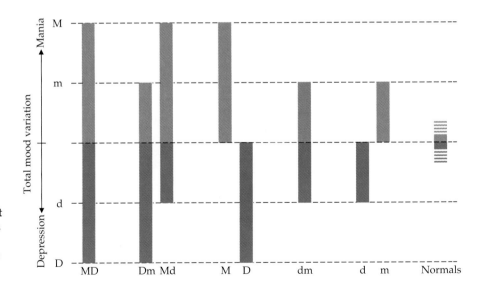

Range of mood variation in normals and in people with different patterns of mood abnormality, as depicted by F. K. Goodwin and K. R. Jamison in *Manic-Depressive Illness* (1990).

cept "mental disorder". . . . In *DSM-III-R* each of the mental disorders is conceptualized as a clinically significant behavioral or psychological syndrome or pattern that occurs in a person and that is associated with present distress (a painful symptom) or disability (impairment in one or more important areas of functioning) or with a significantly increased risk of suffering death, pain, disability, or an important loss of freedom. In addition, this syndrome or pattern must not be merely an expectable response to a particular event, e.g., the death of a loved one. . . . Neither deviant behavior, e.g., political, religious, or sexual, nor conflicts that are primarily between the individual and society are mental disorders unless the deviance or conflict is a symptom of a dysfunction in the person, as described above. . . . There is no assumption that each mental disorder is a discrete entity with sharp boundaries (discontinuity) between it and other mental disorders, or between it and no mental disorder.

DSM-III-R enumerates criteria for the diagnosis of a manic syndrome or a depressive syndrome, as shown in the boxes on the following pages. A mood episode is a mood syndrome that is not due to a known organic factor (e.g., a drug) and is not part of a nonmood psychotic disorder (e.g., schizophrenia). A mood disorder is a specific pattern of mood episodes. Patients who have episodes of mania and episodes of depression are classified as having bipolar disorder (the official term, used because patients swing from one pole of extreme mood to the other) or manic-depressive illness (the popular term). Patients who only become depressed are classified as having major depression (the official term), also called unipolar disorder (since they swing only to the depressive pole).

Mood disorders are remarkably common. Bipolar disorder affects about one person in a hundred, male and female alike, with an average age of onset of about thirty. Major depression is even more common, affecting at least one person in twenty, women twice as often as men, with an average age of onset in the forties. Both disorders are life-threatening, in that between 15 and 20 percent of people with either bipolar disorder or recurrent major depression commit suicide.

The cycling between mania and depression that characterizes bipolar disorder is displayed in a more moderate form by people with a disorder called cyclothymia. The defining characteristics of cyclothymia are numerous mild manic episodes (called hypomanic episodes) that do not impair occupational or social functioning, alternating with numerous periods of mild depression. Since cyclothymia tends to run in the families of patients with bipolar disorder, it is suspected that the two disorders are variants of the same underlying condition. In fact, the same basic cause might give rise to a number of patterns of mood variation, with some at the blurred margins of normality.

Diagnostic Criteria for Manic Episode

Note: A "Manic Syndrome" is defined as including criteria A, B, and C below. A "Hypomanic Syndrome" is defined as including criteria A and B, but not C, i.e., no marked impairment.

A. A distinct period of abnormally and persistently elevated, expansive, or irritable mood.

B. During the period of mood disturbance, at least three of the following symptoms have persisted (four if the mood is only irritable) and have been present to a significant degree:

  (1) inflated self-esteem or grandiosity
  (2) decreased need for sleep, e.g., feels rested after only three hours of sleep
  (3) more talkative than usual or pressure to keep talking
  (4) flight of ideas or subjective experience that thoughts are racing
  (5) distractibility, i.e., attention too easily drawn to unimportant or irrelevant external stimuli
  (6) increase in goal-directed activity (either socially, at work or school, or sexually) or psychomotor agitation

  (7) excessive involvement in pleasurable activities which have a high potential for painful consequences, e.g., the person engages in unrestrained buying sprees, sexual indiscretions, or foolish business investments

C. Mood disturbance sufficiently severe to cause marked impairment in occupational functioning or in usual social activities or relationships with others, or to necessitate hospitalization to prevent harm to self or others.

D. At no time during the disturbance have there been delusions or hallucinations for as long as two weeks in the absence of prominent mood symptoms (i.e., before the mood symptoms developed or after they have remitted).

E. Not superimposed on Schizophrenia.

F. It cannot be established that an organic factor initiated and maintained the disturbance. **Note:** Somatic antidepressant treatment (e.g., drugs, ECT) that apparently precipitates a mood disturbance should not be considered an etiologic organic factor.

Diagnostic criteria from the American Psychiatric Association: *Diagnostic and Statistical Manual of Mental Disorders, Third Edition, Revised,* Washington, D.C., American Psychiatric Association, 1987. Reprinted by permission.

Diagnostic Criteria for Major Depressive Episode

Note: A "Major Depressive Syndrome" is defined as criterion A below.

A. At least five of the following symptoms have been present during the same two-week period and represent a change from previous functioning; at least one of the symptoms is either (1) depressed mood, or (2) loss of interest or pleasure.

   (1) depressed mood (or can be irritable mood in children and adolescents) most of the day, nearly every day, as indicated either by subjective account or observation by others

   (2) markedly diminished interest or pleasure in all, or almost all, activities most of the day, nearly every day (as indicated either by subjective account or observation by others of apathy most of the time)

   (3) significant weight loss or weight gain when not dieting (e.g., more than 5% of body weight in a month), or decrease or increase in appetite nearly every day (in children, consider failure to make expected weight gains)

   (4) insomnia or hypersomnia nearly every day

   (5) psychomotor agitation or retardation nearly every day (observable by others, not merely subjective feelings of restlessness or being slowed down)

   (6) fatigue or loss of energy nearly every day

   (7) feelings of worthlessness or excessive or inappropriate guilt (which may be delusional) nearly every day (not merely self-reproach or guilt about being sick)

   (8) diminished ability to think or concentrate, or indecisiveness, nearly every day (either by subjective account or as observed by others)

   (9) recurrent thoughts of death (not just fear of dying), recurrent suicidal ideation without a specific plan, or a suicide attempt or a specific plan for committing suicide

B. (1) It cannot be established that an organic factor initiated and maintained the disturbance

   (2) The disturbance is not a normal reaction to the death of a loved one (Uncomplicated Bereavement)

Note: Morbid preoccupation with worthlessness, suicidal ideation, marked functional impairment or psychomotor retardation, or prolonged duration suggest bereavement complicated by Major Depression.

C. At no time during the disturbance have there been delusions or hallucinations for as long as two weeks in the absence of prominent mood symptoms (i.e., before the mood symptoms developed or after they have remitted).

D. Not superimposed on Schizophrenia.

Genetics of Mood Disorders

One of the most compelling features of mood disorders, especially bipolar disorder, is, indeed, this tendency to run in families—a fact often observed by biographers and historians. Consider, for example, the Churchill family. It is well known that Winston Churchill suffered from major depression, which he referred to as his "Black Dog." One of his biographers, Lord Moran, recorded the following reminiscence:

> When I was young, for two or three years the lights faded out of the picture. I did my work. I sat in the House of Commons, but black depression settled on me. It helped me to talk to Clemmie about it. I don't like standing near the edge of a platform when an express train is passing through. I like to stand right back and if possible to get a pillar between me and the train. I don't like to stand at the side of a ship and look down into the water. A second's action would end everything.

Winston also frequently revealed a manic side in his periods of exuberant self-confidence and in his indefatigability both as prime minister and as author. So too did Winston's father, Lord Randolph, who swung from

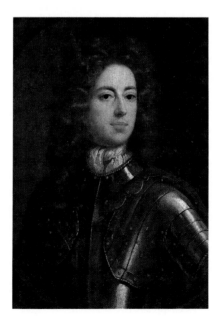 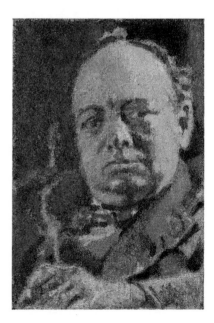

Winston Churchill *(right)* and a famous ancestor, the first Duke of Marlborough *(left)*, two members of a family with a high incidence of mood disorders.

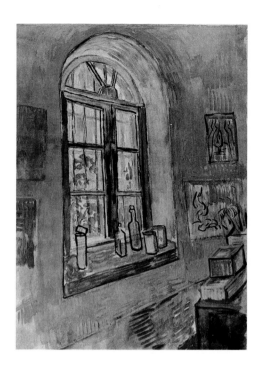

Van Gogh's painting, 1889, of his studio in the asylum in Saint-Rémy.

high mood to low mood in his youth, until his brain was destroyed in the late stages of general paresis. Historians have actually traced the mood disorder in the Churchill family at least as far back as their distinguished ancestor, John Churchill, first Duke of Marlborough (1650–1722). This great English general suffered from intense depression, and there is evidence that his father (named Winston) may have also been affected with a mood disorder.

Another example is the family of Vincent van Gogh. Although the exact nature of van Gogh's affliction is currently controversial, the evidence strongly suggests that he had a form of bipolar disorder. This brilliant artist often produced one masterpiece a day during what were probably intense manic episodes. These periods alternated with severe depressive episodes, sometimes accompanied by psychotic manifestations, including an irrational fear of persecution and disturbed visual perceptions. During one depressive episode, van Gogh must have lapsed into a particularly bizarre mental state (which is not uncommon in patients with bipolar disorder), since he proceeded to cut off part of his right ear. This led to a long period of hospitalization in an asylum in Saint-Rémy, where van Gogh showed great improvement and continued to paint. But when severe depression recurred, he shot himself and died.

Incidence of bipolar disorder and major depression in the general population and in first-degree relatives of a series of patients who had either bipolar disorder or major depression.

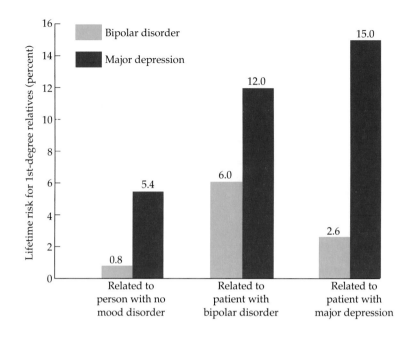

The reason for suspecting that van Gogh's condition sprang from a genetic predisposition is that he had siblings who showed evidence suggestive of mood disorders. His siblings included a brother, Cornelius, who also committed suicide, and a sister, Wilhelmina, who spent decades hospitalized with a disabling psychiatric disorder. Theo, the brother who supported Vincent throughout his life, also had recurrent periods of severe depression.

Of course, to establish convincingly that mood disorders are familial, it is necessary to rely on direct interviews and formal diagnostic criteria rather than on the subjective impressions of biographers. In the past decade, several large systematic studies have, indeed, established that first-degree relatives (parents, children, and siblings) of patients with major depression or bipolar disorder are at markedly greater risk for mood disorder than people without affected relatives. For first-degree relatives of patients with bipolar disorder, the risk of developing this condition is about eight times normal (considerably more in some studies), and the risk of developing major depression is about twice normal. For first-degree relatives of patients with major depression, the risk of developing either major depression or bipolar disorder is about three times normal.

However, even these systematic studies do not establish that mood disorders are genetically transmitted, since the results might be due to

Chapter 6

shared environment rather than to shared genes. One way of testing an environmental explanation is to compare the incidence of mood disorders in identical twins (who share all their genes) with same-sex fraternal twins (who share only half their genes). Only twins who have been raised together since birth and presumably have experienced essentially the same environment are considered; thus, the only major distinction between the identical and fraternal twins is their different degrees of genetic similarity. The results of such studies show that if one identical twin has bipolar disorder, the other twin has a 79 percent chance of developing a major mood disorder (either bipolar disorder or major depression) during his or her lifetime. In contrast, a fraternal twin of a patient with bipolar disorder has only a 24 percent chance of developing a major mood disorder. Although this too is quite a substantial risk, it really is not much greater than the risk that any first-degree relative of a patient with bipolar disorder will develop a major mood disorder, which is about 18 percent.

In Search of the Abnormal Genes

The evidence for genetic factors in mood disorders provided by family and twin studies has encouraged a search for the abnormal gene or genes. The approach now being taken has already been used successfully to find the single gene responsible for each of a number of genetic disorders. It begins with a search for the rough location of the gene that causes a disease, which is ascertained by determining its proximity to a series of several hundred chromosomal markers equally spaced throughout the 24 different chromosomes, as described in Chapter 3. If the precise chromosomal location of a particular marker is known, and a mood disorder is invariably transmitted along with the marker, then the gene responsible for the mood disorder must be very close to the marker. From that point, other techniques may be brought to bear to localize the gene precisely and then identify it.

Given the powerful and continuously improving technology for gene searching, the only other indispensable ingredient is a sufficient number of families with a sufficient number of affected members. On the face of it, such families would seem fairly easy to identify because mood disorders are so prevalent. But the problem is complicated by the possibility of genetic heterogeneity, as mentioned in Chapter 2. Just as the syndrome of anemia might be caused by several different genetic abnormalities (e.g.,

Members of the Old Order Amish community.

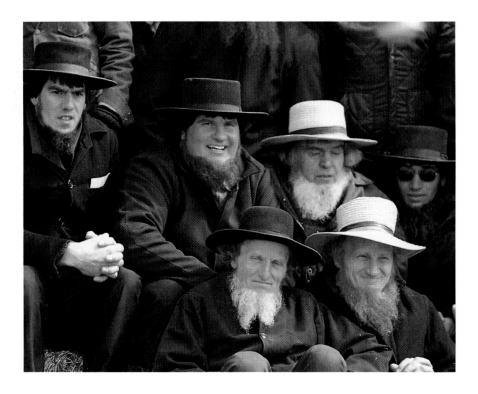

sickle-cell anemia, beta-thalassemia, or hereditary spherocytosis), so too could there be more than one genetic basis for a mood disorder.

Because of the problem of genetic heterogeneity, some investigators have decided to study mood disorders in populations that are geographically or culturally isolated (and whose members therefore only marry other members of the same population) in the hope that all the affected members are descended from a single affected ancestor (and would therefore have the same form of the genetic abnormality). This approach was successfully used in an isolated village in Venezuela to identify the chromosomal location of the gene that causes Huntington's disease. In that case, the affected ancestor could actually be identified; however, because mood disorders are vastly more prevalent than Huntington's disease, even an isolated population could have multiple affected ancestors who might have introduced more than one genetic form of a mood disorder.

Despite these limitations, there are advantages to working with isolated populations, such as the Old Order Amish of Pennsylvania, a closely

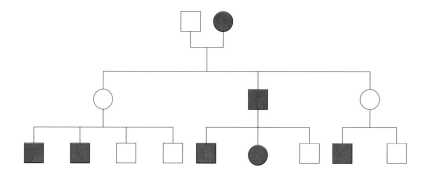

Mood disorders in a fragment of a large Amish pedigree. Affected individuals fulfill the diagnostic criteria for either bipolar disorder or major depression.

knit group whose members seldom leave or marry outside their own community. For one thing, their isolation facilitates examination and identification of family members over several generations. Another advantage is that the Old Order Amish do not use alcohol or other drugs that may give rise to disturbances that can be confused with mood disorders.

Although the Old Order Amish have about the same incidence of mood disorders as the rest of humanity, pedigrees with a very high incidence of bipolar disorder and major depression have been identified. As with the family studies described earlier, both forms of mood disorder are found within a single pedigree. This finding raises the question of whether one should assume that, within a pedigree, both bipolar disorder and major depression are necessarily manifestations of the same abnormal gene. Should work begin with the assumption that in such pedigrees only those with bipolar disorder definitely have the abnormal gene to be searched for, and those with major depression, which has a much greater overall prevalence, may not? In pedigrees with many cases of bipolar disorder, should people with cyclothymia be considered to have the same abnormal gene? If the criteria are too exclusive, it becomes more difficult to find pedigrees with enough affected members to permit statistically significant conclusions. If the criteria are insufficiently exclusive, there is the danger of mixing apples and oranges.

At present, it seems most promising to confine attention to patients who display full-blown bipolar disorder because the evidence for a genetic cause is strongest for this condition. Given the constantly improving techniques for genetic studies, there is reason to be optimistic that a gene or genes that cause bipolar disorder will be discovered within the next decade. Identification of an abnormal gene will then help determine the degree of genetic heterogeneity of bipolar disorder and its relationship to cyclothymia and major depression.

Drugs, Monoamines, and Depression

Although the ultimate genetic cause of mood disorders remains obscure, a great deal has already been learned about the nature of the neurotransmitters that influence mood. We owe this knowledge to studies of the effects of drugs that alter mood; but success in developing effective therapeutic drugs does not mean that we understand the underlying abnormality that leads to the mood extremes. Instead, each drug may be to mood what aspirin is to fever—an agent that alters the expression of an undesirable physiological response without addressing its cause.

The most important discovery to date is that drugs that influence neurotransmission involving one or more of three brain monoamine neurotransmitters—norepinephrine, dopamine, and serotonin—can influence mood. Some of the early studies that led to this general conclusion were described in the previous chapter. As we saw, monoamine oxidase inhibitors, which block the degradation of all these neurotransmitters, alleviate depression. So too does imipramine, which prolongs the synaptic action of these monoamines by blocking the transporters that remove them from the synaptic cleft. Additional early support came from the observation that reserpine, which depletes all three monoamines, induced major depression in about 15 percent of people who took it as a treatment for hypertension. Taken together, these findings strongly support the conclusion that increased monoamine neurotransmission is correlated with good mood.

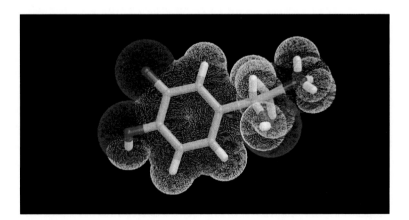

A computer-generated model of norepinephrine.

These early discoveries were followed by many attempts to determine whether the antidepressant drugs exerted their therapeutic effect by acting on only one of the amine neurotransmitters, and if so, which one. Early studies tended to favor the importance of the catecholamines norepinephrine and dopamine. One relevant finding was the reversal of reserpine-induced depression by an amino acid derivative called DOPA, which is a building block of both dopamine and norepinephrine. DOPA increases catecholamine biosynthesis, thereby helping replace the norepinephrine and dopamine that reserpine had depleted, but it does not help replace the depleted serotonin. This finding suggested that depleted catecholamines, rather than depleted serotonin, caused reserpine-induced depression. The action of another amino acid derivative, called AMPT, which inhibits catecholamine biosynthesis (but not serotonin biosynthesis) and aggravates depression, added weight to this opinion. So too did demonstration of the antidepressant effect of desipramine, a derivative of imipramine, which very effectively blocks synaptic reuptake of norepinephrine but has no effect on reuptake of serotonin.

Work with newer antidepressants has recently shifted attention back to serotonin. For example, fluoxetine (marketed under the trade name Prozac) selectively blocks synaptic reuptake of serotonin but does not block reuptake of catecholamines. Fluoxetine has enjoyed tremendous popularity not because it is a better antidepressant than imipramine but because it does not cause certain annoying side effects. Other new antidepressants, such as sertraline and fluvoxamine, also selectively block serotonin reuptake and offer similar advantages, but none is without side effects of its own.

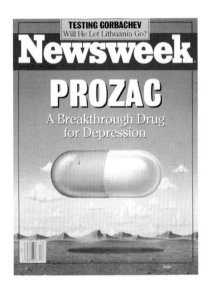

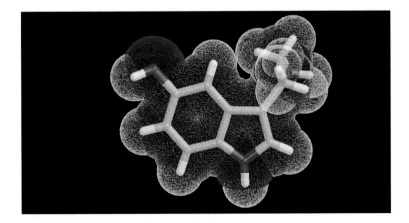

A computer-generated model of serotonin.

Tranylcypromine

Desipramine

At first glance, it seems very difficult to reconcile the evidence that drugs that selectively affect either catecholamines or serotonin influence mood. The most reasonable interpretation is that mood is controlled by neuronal circuits that receive converging neuronal inputs that employ different monoamine neurotransmitters. Augmenting the action of any one of these monoamines might influence this hypothetical neuronal circuit, thereby producing a change in mood.

But this simple view does not fully explain the therapeutic action of the antidepressant drugs, since it fails to address the cause of the lag between the beginning of treatment and the development of a therapeutic response. With all of the drugs currently used, the antidepressant action is usually not apparent for at least ten days after onset of treatment and may not reach its peak for several weeks. Yet all of them, whether they are reuptake blockers or monoamine oxidase inhibitors, influence neurotransmission within hours of administration. Why, then, must so much time pass before the antidepressant action is observed? Do these drugs produce other therapeutically relevant changes in the brain that take weeks to develop?

One consequence of sustained administration of imipramine to experimental animals is actually a gradual reduction in the amounts of particular

Fluoxetine

Effect of Four Commonly Used Antidepressants on Neurotransmission by Norepinephrine and Serotonin

| | | NEUROTRANSMISSION | |
DRUG	ACUTE EFFECT	NOREPINEPHRINE	SEROTONIN
Tranylcypromine	Blocks monoamine oxidase	↑	↑
Imipramine	Blocks norepinephrine and serotonin transporters	↑	↑
Desipramine	Blocks norepinephrine transporter	↑	No change
Fluoxetine	Blocks serotonin transporter	No change	↑

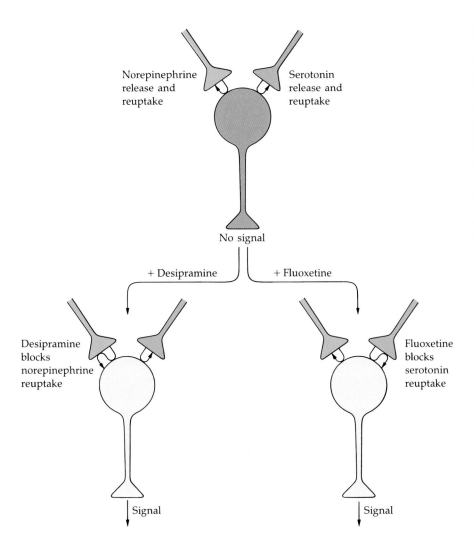

Norepinephrine release and reuptake

Serotonin release and reuptake

No signal

+ Desipramine

+ Fluoxetine

Desipramine blocks norepinephrine reuptake

Fluoxetine blocks serotonin reuptake

Signal

Signal

If a hypothetical mood-controlling neuron is stimulated by a neuron that releases norepinephrine and another neuron that releases serotonin, drugs that prolong the synaptic action of either monoamine may cause the mood-controlling neuron to be activated (symbolized by a change from blue to yellow) and to transmit a signal that elevates mood. This could be the reason that drugs that augment the action of either of these neurotransmitters may have the same net stimulatory effect on mood.

classes of receptors for norepinephrine and serotonin in particular populations of postsynaptic cells. This change, which occurs over the course of several weeks, probably reflects adaptation by neurons that are overstimulated by the elevated monoamine levels induced by imipramine's persistent effect. Presumably, these neurons reduce the number of postsynaptic receptors in order to cut down the stimulation. Unfortunately, there is no persuasive evidence that such reduction has anything to do with the antidepressant effect. Since drugs may set in motion a very complex series of neuronal changes, as discussed in Chapter 5, identification of the one clinically relevant change may prove to be exceptionally challenging.

Cortisol and Depression

CH₂OH structure label area

Cortisol

Monoamine neurotransmitters are not the only molecules whose actions have been correlated with a depressed state: There is also a great deal of evidence relating disturbances in cortisol levels with depression. Cortisol is a hormone produced by the adrenal cortex, from which it is released in large amounts in response to stress. Transported by the bloodstream, it alters the metabolic activity of many different cells throughout the body. By binding to glucocorticoid receptors (discussed in Chapter 3), cortisol can influence the expression of a number of genes in the brain and other tissues, and this altered expression, in turn, produces many of the physiological changes we develop in response to sustained stress.

It has been known for many years that high blood levels of cortisol may be associated with depression. For example, people with Cushing's syndrome, which is caused by diseases that markedly increase cortisol secretion, often are depressed. Likewise, patients given large doses of cortisol as treatment for arthritis or allergic reactions may also show depressive symptoms. In these people, the elevated cortisol levels apparently are a cause of the depression.

These are not, however, the only instances of depression associated with high cortisol levels. Many patients who suffer from major depression have high levels of blood cortisol that appear to be a consequence, rather than a cause, of the depressive syndrome. This finding is very surprising because cortisol levels are normally carefully regulated by a series of feedback systems involving the anterior pituitary gland and the brain, which are both involved in controlling secretion of cortisol by the adrenal cortex.

That many patients with major depression have elevated blood cortisol levels suggests a correlation between an abnormality in the cortisol feedback system and the depressive state. We know the abnormality is not permanent, because people who recover from major depression generally have normal cortisol levels. Apparently, therefore, the primary (and unknown) abnormality in depression leads to a transient failure of a component of the cortisol feedback system, which allows cortisol levels to remain too high. However, since high levels of cortisol can cause depression independently of feedback failures, it is possible that once cortisol blood levels become elevated in depressed patients, the high levels may perpetuate the depressed state.

Treating Mania

In the previous chapter, we saw how the treatment of depression was revolutionized in the 1950s by chance observations of the antidepressant effects of iproniazid and imipramine. Serendipity also played an important role in revolutionizing the treatment of mania. The critical discovery was made in 1948 by John Cade, an Australian psychiatrist who was searching for a toxic agent in the urine of manic patients by injecting guinea pigs with urine samples and observing the behavioral effects. Cade also examined the behavioral effects of normal urinary constituents, including uric acid salts. Since lithium urate is the most soluble uric acid salt, Cade used it in his experiments. He found that guinea pigs injected with lithium urate became lethargic. Since lithium carbonate produced the same effect, he concluded that the lithium, rather than the urate, was responsible.

Cade then decided to treat a manic patient with lithium salts. Amazingly, it worked. Writing in 1970, Cade recalled this decision and its results:

> It may seem a long way from lethargy in guinea pigs to the control of manic excitement, but as these investigations had commenced in an attempt to demonstrate some possibly excreted toxin in the urine of manic patients, the association of ideas is explicable. As lithium salts had been in use in medical practice since the middle of the nineteenth century, albeit in a haphazard way with negligible therapeutic results, there seemed no ethical contraindications to using them in mania, especially as single and repeated doses of lithium citrate and lithium carbonate in the doses contemplated produced no discernible ill effects on the investigator himself.
>
> . . . [Y]ou may be interested in the case report of the very first manic patient ever deliberately and successfully treated with lithium salts. This was a little wizened man of 51 who had been in a state of chronic manic excitement for five years. He was amiably restless, dirty, destructive, mischievous and interfering. He had enjoyed preeminent nuisance value in a back ward for all those years and bid fair to remain there for the rest of his life.

He commenced treatment with lithium citrate 1200 mg tid* on 29 March, 1948. On the fourth day, the optimistic therapist thought he saw some change for the better but acknowledged that it could have been his expectant imagination; the nursing staff were non-committal but loyal. However, by the fifth day it was clear that he was in fact more settled, tidier, less disinhibited and less distractible. From then on there was steady improvement so that in three weeks he was enjoying the unaccustomed and quite unexpected amenities of a convalescent ward. As he had been ill so long and confined to a chronic ward he found normal surroundings and liberty of movement strange at first. Owing to this, as well as housing difficulties and the necessity of determining a satisfactory maintenance dose, he was kept under observation for two months. He remained perfectly well and left hospital on 9 July, 1948, on indefinite leave with instructions to take a maintenance dose of lithium carbonate, 300 mg bid†.

Despite their dramatic nature, Cade's results, which were published in *The Medical Journal of Australia* in 1949, did not attract much attention until the Danish psychiatrists Mogens Schou and Poul Baastrup replicated and extended his findings. Schou and Baastrup observed that sustained administration of lithium not only prevented the recurrence of manic attacks but also prevented the recurrent depressions of patients with bipolar disorder. This action of lithium may be contrasted with those of other treatments for mania and depression in bipolar patients, which act on monoamine systems. For example, chlorpromazine, which calms manic excitement by blocking monoamine receptors, may, in the process, induce depression; and antidepressants that augment monoamine function (e.g., imipramine) often provoke a manic episode. That lithium has antidepressant as well as antimanic effects is both wonderful and puzzling.

These paradoxical effects of lithium may be the result of its effect on second messenger systems involved in neuromodulation. For example, in the low doses needed for therapeutic action, lithium significantly inhibits an enzyme known as inositol phosphatase, which controls the breakdown of inositol phosphates to inositol. Normally, the inositol so produced is then reused to regenerate the plasma membrane phospholipid PIP_2, which is, as we have seen, the precursor of two second messengers, diacylglycerol (DAG) and inositol trisphosphate (IP_3), both of which are involved in

---

*Three times a day.

†Two times a day.

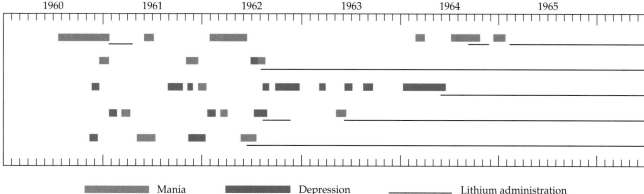

1960	1961	1962	1963	1964	1965

Mania ▬▬▬ Depression ▬▬▬ Lithium administration ▬▬▬

Effect of lithium treatment on periods of mania or depression in five patients.

modulation of postsynaptic membrane properties. Since lithium makes inositol unavailable, PIP_2 is not regenerated, and IP_3 and DAG cannot be released to act as second messengers. In this way, lithium inhibits this form of neuromodulation. It has been speculated that lithium's ability to temper mood swings toward either pole may result from attenuation of hyperactive neuromodulation mechanisms involved in both mania and depression.

Lithium's therapeutic activity could also be due to another known effect on neuromodulation. At levels used to treat patients with bipolar disorder, lithium has been shown to directly influence neuronal regulatory mechanisms employing G proteins and protein kinases. These effects might also damp major mood oscillations in either direction.

In addition to lithium, two other drugs, carbamazepine and valproic acid, have been found useful in the treatment of manic patients. Both these antimanic drugs happen to be anticonvulsants as well and are effective in preventing the uncontrollable neuronal activity that results in epileptic seizures. How their anticonvulsant effects are related to their efficacy in ameliorating manic episodes is not known.

Carbamazepine

Valproic acid

Electroconvulsive Therapy

Also a mystery is the mechanism of action of the most potent known antidepressant treatment, electroconvulsive therapy. This treatment, which amounts to deliberately inducing an electrical seizure in the brain, was introduced in the 1930s for the management of psychotic behavior. Initially, it was administered without anesthesia or muscle relaxants, so that the patient made violent movements during the seizures, that sometimes resulted in bone fractures. Because of this serious side effect, electroconvulsive therapy fell into disfavor when potent pharmacological agents to manage mood disorders became available in the 1950s.

Electroconvulsive therapy has been receiving renewed attention in recent years for the management of severe depression that is refractory to pharmacological treatment. Patients are now given a general anesthetic so that they are not conscious during the actual procedure, and they also receive a powerful muscle relaxant so that the seizure in the brain is not accompanied by significant body movements. One potentially serious side effect of repeated treatments is that the patient may show memory impairment, especially for events that immediately preceded the seizure. However, with the small number of treatments generally sufficient to alleviate depression, there is no significant impairment of subsequent learning.

In a very large percentage of cases, electroconvulsive therapy brings about rapid clearing of depression, without the long time lag characteristic of antidepressant drugs. A single treatment sometimes has substantial effects, and half a dozen treatments may be all that is needed to return the patient to a completely normal mood state. Since any inclination to suicide generally disappears promptly, electroconvulsive therapy is often life-saving.

Given the complex effects that an induced brain seizure must have on neuronal functions, it is little wonder that we do not understand how such seizures alleviate depression. An extreme perturbation like electroconvulsive therapy provokes molecular changes too diverse to be untangled and correlated to mood states by any experimental approach now available. It must be emphasized, however, that electroconvulsive therapy should not be withheld from patients whose life may depend on it simply because we do not understand how it works.

Future Directions

It is generally accepted that development of effective treatments for mania and depression represents one of the great practical advances in psychiatry over the past generation. Appropriate pharmacological intervention produces dramatic effects in most patients. Cognitive therapy, a form of structured psychotherapy that is designed to overcome negative views of oneself and of one's future, has also greatly assisted patients with severe mood disorders to lead relatively normal lives.

Because of the power of these treatments, the National Institute of Mental Health has mounted a campaign to promote public awareness of the prevalence of mood disorders. Its goal is to encourage the treatment of the vast number of people with mood disorders who have not yet sought professional help. It is my hope that readers of this book will play a role in helping some of those who would benefit from treatment to seek and receive it.

It should also be apparent from reading this chapter, however, that success in treatment has been achieved despite a very limited understanding of the underlying pathology of mood disorders. Finding the primary defects responsible for mood disorders may be particularly difficult because abnormal mood syndromes may have numerous potential causes. For this reason, genetic research is especially promising. With new techniques, even the challenging problem of possible genetic heterogeneity of mood disorders should eventually prove tractable.

Advances in drug therapy will also continue, guided in part by our growing knowledge of the structure and special properties of various neurotransmitter receptors as well by similar work with the transporter proteins involved in reuptake of neurotransmitters into synaptic terminals. The cloning of cDNAs for many receptors and transporters, which allows these proteins to be studied in isolation, may facilitate the development of new pharmacological agents with specific affinities for one or another of them.

All in all, work on molecular aspects of mood disorders has a bright future. There is much we need to learn; but reasonably effective tools are in hand.

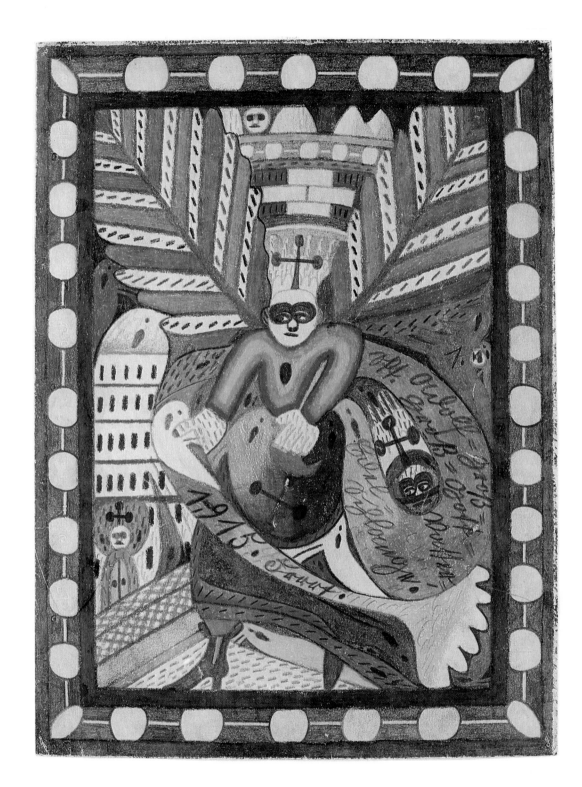

7

SCHIZOPHRENIA

All of us have an empathic understanding of mood extremes because we have experienced these states, at least in muted form. Though it may be difficult to appreciate how black a depressed patient's mood really is or how frenzied a manic patient may become, neither depression nor mania strikes us as innately strange or incomprehensible.

This is not the case with schizophrenia. Patients with this disorder behave in ways that normal people find very difficult to understand. Its incomprehensibility is vividly illustrated by the reaction of a small group of second-year medical students as they and their instructor interview their first schizophrenic patient.

Sitting with them is a young person about their own age, who speaks clearly and intelligently. He has agreed to the interview because he is quite willing to tell them his story, which starts out very much as would any of

OPPOSITE: *Saint-Adolf-Grand-Grand-God-Father*, 1915,
———— by Adolf Wölfli (1864–1930), who at 31 was hospi- ————
talized with symptoms of schizophrenia.

143

theirs. But before long, without any prodding, he is talking about the FBI. He firmly believes that the FBI has assembled a special team (partly a SWAT team) whose mission is to find evidence so that they can arrest him. For what crime? He looks away, smiles, but will not say. What evidence does he have for this belief? He has a warning voice in his head that says "there is one." Is the voice real? Of course.

The initial reaction of the students to this interview is that the so-called patient is either a skillful liar or a hired actor. This is not a disheveled homeless person whose strange behavior on the street has attracted their passing glances; surely nobody who seems so much like them could believe such crazy nonsense. They are incredulous. Such is the nature of schizophrenia.

Characteristics and Incidence of Schizophrenia

Like mood disorders, schizophrenia is identified on the basis of a pattern of abnormal behaviors. The most characteristic of these behaviors are false beliefs (called delusions) and abnormal perceptions (called hallucinations), which reflect a failure to differentiate inner preconceptions and expectations from data coming from the outside world. This inability to distinguish what is real from what is not is a hallmark of psychosis, a loosely defined term for a state that is characteristic of (but not synonymous with) schizophrenia.

Patients with schizophrenia may hear voices that seem to be warning them or attempting to control them (auditory hallucinations), may smell nonexistent smells (olfactory hallucinations), or may see apparitions such as devils (visual hallucinations). They may be convinced that they are the victims of organized plots by powerful adversaries (persecutory delusions) or that radio waves or laser beams are focused on their brains, generating unwelcome but uncontrollable thoughts (delusions of being controlled). Like Adolf Wölfli, whose drawing opens this chapter, they also may withdraw into a world of their own that is peopled with fictional characters and may become detached from their real surroundings. Their speech may become disorganized, incomprehensible, and bizarre.

This dramatic and disabling condition is not rare: it is estimated that about one in every hundred persons will manifest the specific pattern of symptoms that is necessary for the diagnosis of schizophrenia. Comparably high rates are found not only in the United States and Western Europe but also in nations as diverse as India and Japan. Men and women are affected about equally; however, men tend to develop the disorder at an earlier age, often before they are 20 years old, whereas about one third of affected women do not display psychotic behavior until they are past 30. Moreover, although schizophrenia may be more visible today among certain groups, such as the urban poor, it is prevalent among all classes.

Schizophrenia is a very expensive disorder. The National Institute of Mental Health estimates that in the United States alone the cost of care and the income lost together amount to about $50 billion a year. In addition to this great financial drain, schizophrenia is socially costly, devastating families and accounting for about a third of the nation's homeless. It is also life-threatening, leading to suicide in about 10 percent of cases.

The reason why schizophrenia is such a huge financial and social problem is that it strikes young people and renders them nonproductive and troublesome for the many remaining decades of their lives. Parents feel guilty, ashamed, helpless; society recognizes the tragedy but shudders at the cost.

Variants of Schizophrenia

Studies of the incidence of schizophrenia are, of course, predicated on the notion that the condition can be reliably defined. Unfortunately, this is only approximately true; people who are lumped together as having schizophrenia vary greatly with respect to both the nature of their symptoms and the expression of those symptoms throughout the course of their lives.

For Emil Kraepelin (1856–1926), a German psychiatrist who made important contributions to the classification of mental illness beginning in the late nineteenth century, a defining characteristic of this psychotic condition was that it had a deteriorating course. In fact, he applied the Latin term *dementia praecox* (literally, "premature dementia," that is, affecting the young rather than the old) to describe the disease. Like many of his predecessors, Kraepelin believed that the underlying basis of dementia praecox was probably brain deterioration. He considered manic-depressive illness (a term that he used) to be fundamentally different, in that it allowed periods of recovery and normal mental functioning.

Emil Kraepelin.

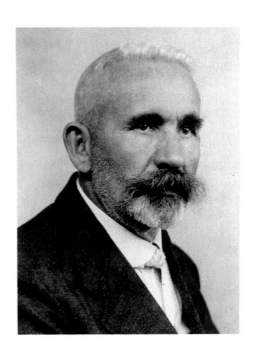

Led by his observations of patients with a different pattern of illness, the Swiss psychiatrist Eugen Bleuler (1857–1939) came to an alternative conclusion. In Bleuler's view, these patients had split (schizo-) minds (-phrenia); accordingly, he coined the term schizophrenia in 1911 to emphasize that those afflicted with this form of the disorder could function normally at certain times. That mental function could be recovered at all suggested that the condition resulted from a transient physiological abnormality of the brain rather than from permanent brain degeneration.

In *DSM-III-R*, the diagnosis of schizophrenia includes many different types of patients, including those with the features emphasized by Kraepelin and Bleuler. Although many schizophrenic patients may progressively deteriorate into the withdrawn state that Kraepelin described, this is not a defining characteristic of schizophrenia; Bleuler's patients, who could improve or recover, are also in this category.

DSM-III-R then breaks down the umbrella category of schizophrenia into various types, including two common and distinctive ones—paranoid and disorganized. The essential feature of the paranoid type is preoccupation with one or more systematized delusions, usually coupled with frequent auditory hallucinations related to a single theme. Such patients may function reasonably well when they are not acting on the basis of these

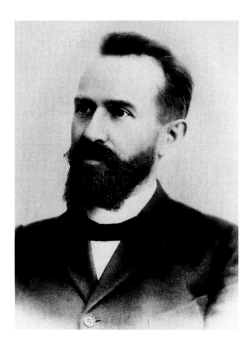
Eugen Bleuler.

disordered thoughts and perceptions. In contrast, the essential feature of the disorganized type is incoherent behavior that an observer has trouble interpreting, combined with an extreme paucity of emotional expression. These patients usually have fragmentary delusions or hallucinations as well, but the content is not systematized into a coherent theme. The outlook for patients with disorganized-type schizophrenia is especially grim: extreme social impairment, without significant remission, is common.

DSM-III-R also recognizes two other major types of schizophrenia. The catatonic type, common in Kraepelin and Bleuler's time, but now extremely rare, is characterized by abnormal posturing, stupor, and mutism. The undifferentiated type is characterized by a mixture of symptoms.

To complicate matters, some patients display both psychotic symptoms and symptoms of a mood disorder. Such patients are subdivided into two categories according to whether the psychotic and affective symptoms are expressed together or separately. If a patient reports having delusions or hallucinations *during* periods of severe mood disturbance, the diagnosis is mood disorder with psychotic features. If delusions or hallucinations are expressed for at least two weeks *in the absence of* severe mood disturbance, the patient is placed into yet another category, called schizoaffective disorder.

Diagnostic Criteria for Schizophrenia

A. Presence of characteristic psychotic symptoms in the active phase: either (1), (2), or (3) for at least one week (unless the symptoms are successfully treated):

   (1) two of the following:
      (a) delusions
      (b) prominent hallucinations (throughout the day for several days or several times a week for several weeks, each hallucinatory experience not being limited to a few brief moments)
      (c) incoherence or marked loosening of associations
      (d) catatonic behavior
      (e) flat or grossly inappropriate affect

   (2) bizarre delusions (i.e., involving a phenomenon that the person's culture would regard as totally implausible, e.g., thought broadcasting, being controlled by a dead person)

   (3) prominent hallucinations [as defined in (1)(b) above] of a voice with content having no apparent relation to depression or elation, or a voice keeping up a running commentary on the person's behavior or thoughts, or two or more voices conversing with each other

B. During the course of the disturbance, functioning in such areas as work, social relations, and self-care is markedly below the highest level achieved before onset of the disturbance (or, when the onset is in childhood or adolescence, failure to achieve expected level of social development).

C. Schizoaffective Disorder and Mood Disorder with Psychotic Features have been ruled out, i.e., if a Major Depressive or Manic Syndrome has ever been present during an active phase of the disturbance, the total duration of all episodes of a mood syndrome has been brief relative to the total duration of the active and residual phases of the disturbance.

D. Continuous signs of the disturbance for at least six months. The six-month period must include an active phase (of at least one week, or less if symptoms have been successfully treated) during which there

---

The reason for all these categories is that they provide a shorthand for communication, guide treatment selection, and shape expectations about the patient's long-term prognosis. At present, however, we have no idea whether the different categories of schizophrenia are due to the same cause or different ones or, for that matter, whether a single category might have different causes. For now, our best clue to what causes schizophrenia is that many of those affected seem to have inherited it.

were psychotic symptoms characteristic of Schizophrenia (symptoms in A), with or without a prodromal or residual phase, as defined below.

Prodromal phase: A clear deterioration in functioning before the active phase of the disturbance that is not due to a disturbance in mood or to a Psychoactive Substance Use Disorder and that involves at least two of the symptoms listed below.

Residual phase: Following the active phase of the disturbance, persistence of at least two of the symptoms noted below, these not being due to a disturbance in mood or to a Psychoactive Substance Use Disorder.

Prodromal or Residual Symptoms:

(1) marked social isolation or withdrawal
(2) marked impairment in role functioning as wage-earner, student, or homemaker
(3) markedly peculiar behavior (e.g., collecting garbage, talking to self in public, hoarding food)
(4) marked impairment in personal hygiene and grooming

(5) blunted or inappropriate affect
(6) digressive, vague, overelaborate, or circumstantial speech, or poverty of speech, or poverty of content of speech
(7) odd beliefs or magical thinking, influencing behavior and inconsistent with cultural norms, e.g., superstitiousness, belief in clairvoyance, telepathy, "sixth sense," "others can feel my feelings," overvalued ideas, ideas of reference
(8) unusual perceptual experiences, e.g., recurrent illusions, sensing the presence of a force or person not actually present
(9) marked lack of initiative, interests, or energy.

Examples: Six months of prodromal symptoms with one week of symptoms from A; no prodromal symptoms with six months of symptoms from A; no prodromal symptoms with one week of symptoms from A and six months of residual symptoms.

E. It cannot be established that an organic factor initiated and maintained the disturbance.

Diagnostic criteria from the American Psychiatric Association: *Diagnostic and Statistical Manual of Mental Disorders, Third Edition, Revised*, Washington, D.C., American Psychiatric Association, 1987. Reprinted by permission.

Evidence for a Genetic Basis

Persuasive evidence for a genetic basis for schizophrenia comes from studies correlating the risks for this disorder with the degree of relatedness to an affected individual. In these studies, parents, children, and other relatives are examined for evidence of relevant symptoms, and all variants of

The lifetime risk of developing schizophrenia is correlated with genetic relatedness to a person with schizophrenia.

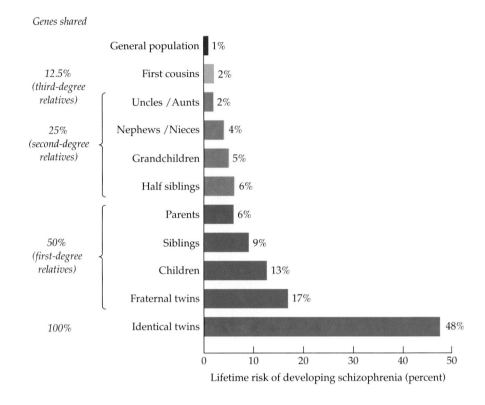

schizophrenia are lumped together. Since schizophrenia, like many genetic disorders, may not appear until advanced adulthood, some of the asymptomatic people interviewed at a young age may manifest the disorder as they grow older. Therefore, extrapolations are made, and the data are expressed as the lifetime risk of displaying sufficient abnormality to justify the diagnosis.

Irving Gottesman at the University of Virginia has summarized evidence for the familial nature of schizophrenia from 40 family and twin studies of European populations examined between 1920 and 1987. The results indicate that, although members of a family also share similar environments, a relative's risk of manifesting schizophrenia increases with the number of genes shared with the schizophrenic person. For example, first-degree relatives (parents, siblings, children), who share 50 percent of the patient's genes, have a higher incidence of schizophrenia than second-degree relatives (uncles, aunts, nephews, nieces, grandchildren), who share only 25 percent. Third-degree relatives (first cousins), who share 12.5 percent of the genes, still have a measurably higher risk than nonrelatives.

The inference from these findings is that the more genes one shares with a schizophrenic person, the higher the probability of sharing the one or few that cause the disorder. This inference is supported by studies comparing the concordance (a term for expression of the same trait in both members of a twin pair) of schizophrenia in identical twin pairs with the concordance in fraternal twin pairs. Identical twins, who share all their genes, show 48 percent concordance, whereas fraternal twins, who share only 50 percent of their genes, show 17 percent concordance. Given that the two members of either type of twin pair ordinarily share the same environment, this finding is strong evidence for a genetic basis for schizophrenia.

It is notable, however, that identical twins do not show complete concordance for schizophrenia. To be sure, their concordance rate is far greater than the 1 percent incidence in the general population and significantly greater than the concordance rate among fraternal twins. But if schizophrenia is caused by an abnormal gene or genes, and all the genes of identical

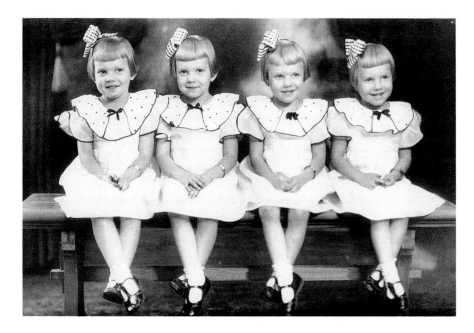

Identical quadruplets (known under the fictitious surname Genain) who each developed symptoms of schizophrenia between the ages of 22 and 24 and who have been repeatedly evaluated at the National Institute of Mental Health since the 1950s. The different form that the disorder has taken in each of them has been taken as evidence for an interaction between predisposing genes and life events.

The effects of penetrance and variable expressivity. All individuals in the same row share an identical gene that has the potential to produce a phenotype, such as a mental illness. In this diagram, the intensity of color is correlated with the intensity of behavioral symptoms.

EXPRESSION OF A TRAIT
(each box represents an individual)

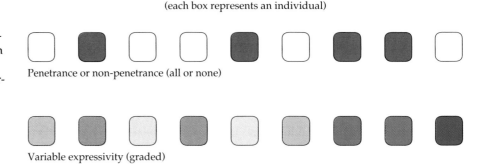

Penetrance or non-penetrance (all or none)

Variable expressivity (graded)

twins are exactly the same, why is their concordance rate only about 50 percent and not 100 percent?

One explanation for this outcome is that genes do not work in isolation. In Chapter 2 we discussed the disorder phenylketonuria, in which abnormal genes are not sufficient to produce the abnormal phenotype, mental retardation. In this case, a known environmental factor, ingestion of phenylalanine, is essential for the expression of the abnormal phenotype. For many other genetic diseases, however, the factors required for expression of the abnormal phenotype have not been identified.

Geneticists have long known that some people with a disease gene (verifiable by direct DNA examination) show either no evidence of the disease, a phenomenon called nonpenetrance, or a range of expression of the disease gene (from mild to severe), a phenomenon called variable expressivity. Variable expressivity is very common. For example, the gene for the autosomal dominant disorder called von Recklinghausen's disease is variably expressed: in certain affected members of a family, the only manifestations are barely detectable brownish spots on the skin, whereas in other, less fortunate, relatives, monstrous and grotesque facial and body deformities result. The extent to which the disease gene is expressed in a particular person is presumed to be influenced by unknown environmental factors as well as by other genes.

Inherited mental illnesses may also show nonpenetrance and variable expressivity. The latter is suggested by family studies of patients with schizophrenia, which frequently identify many family members who exhibit suspiciousness, odd thought patterns, and a tendency to be withdrawn, traits that appear to be related to (though by no means sufficient for a diagnosis of) schizophrenia. Identical twins of patients with schizophrenia sometimes manifest behavior that would justify a *DSM-III-R* diagnosis of schizoid personality disorder or schizotypal personality disorder, suggesting that even if a twin pair is formally scored as being discordant (a term for expression of a trait in only one member of a twin pair) for schizophrenia, the mildly affected twin may still be expressing the same gene or genes that cause full-blown psychosis in the sibling.

Another explanation for discordance of some identical twin pairs for schizophrenia is that the affected twin's schizophrenia may be due to environmental factors. There is no evidence that psychological factors, such as the behavior of parents, is responsible for this discordance, but evidence from recent studies of brain structure in 15 pairs of identical twins discordant for schizophrenia suggests that brain infection or injury may contribute to the development of the condition in the affected twin.

In these studies, brain structure was examined by means of a technique called magnetic resonance imaging, which provides images of different levels of the brain and can distinguish brain tissue from fluids that fill certain internal cavities called ventricles. Normally, identical twins are alike in the detailed structural features of their brains. In 12 of the 15 twin pairs discordant for schizophrenia, however, the affected twin showed evidence of some degree of abnormal brain structure. In some instances, the schizophrenic twin had a striking enlargement of the brain ventricles, presumably reflecting degenerative shrinkage of the brain tissue surrounding them. The observation that only the schizophrenic twin had this structural abnormality suggests that an environmental factor caused brain damage,

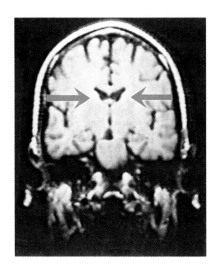 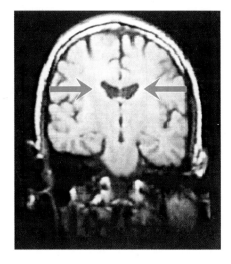

Abnormal brain structure associated with schizophrenia as indicated by magnetic resonance imaging scans of the brains of a pair of identical twins only one of whom is schizophrenic. In this case the twin on the right (who has schizophrenia) has much larger ventricles (dark butterfly-shaped cavities), indicating a loss of brain tissue.

which played an essential role in the development of the pattern of psychotic behavior.

Despite this evidence that environmental factors contribute to the development of schizophrenia in some patients, our best hope for progress is to intensify the search for the genes that also play an essential role. What makes genetic studies so timely is that, given favorable pedigrees, current gene mapping techniques should be up to the task of identifying the relevant gene or genes, even in the face of the problems of genetic heterogeneity and polygenic inheritance. In contrast, there are at present no leads to the environmental factors that cause schizophrenia and no strategy for their identification. Although some forms of schizophrenia may well prove to be of environmental rather than genetic origin, positive identification of even one gene that leads to schizophrenia will have a profound effect on our subsequent approach to this disorder.

Drug-Induced Psychosis

Genetic studies seek the ultimate biological causes of schizophrenia, that is, the abnormal gene or genes that result in a fundamental disturbance in brain function. While this search proceeds, other approaches are also being taken to identify the abnormalities underlying schizophrenia. Since a number of drugs produce changes in thoughts and perceptions reminiscent of those displayed by schizophrenic patients, an understanding of their effects could lead to insights into the causes of schizophrenic symptoms. Most remarkable, perhaps, is the finding that drugs with different primary modes of action can produce similar symptoms, which bolsters the case for the view that the naturally occurring disease has multiple causes.

Enormous interest in drug-induced perceptual changes was stimulated by the widespread use of the potent hallucinogen lysergic acid diethylamide (LSD), which began in the 1950s. LSD is made by modifying a chemical derived from a fungus that infects grains. Its hallucinogenic properties were discovered in 1943, quite by chance, when the Swiss chemist Albert Hofmann accidentally ingested minute quantities of a batch of the drug he was in the process of synthesizing. Hofmann noted especially striking visual perceptual distortions, including changes in the shape of common objects and vividly colored hallucinations. The experience was thrilling but also somewhat terrifying, not only to Hofmann but to many of those who have taken this drug since then.

LSD's chemical structure also has aroused considerable interest because embedded within it is an indole ring like that of the neurotransmitter serotonin. An indole ring is also present in psilocybin, the active hallucinogenic ingredient in certain psychedelic mushrooms, and in dimethyltryptamine, a totally synthetic hallucinogen. Since each of these drugs has also been shown to interact with certain serotonin receptors, it seems likely that the hallucinogenic experience involves alteration of serotonin's functions, though the details have not been worked out.

Whereas hallucinogens like LSD produce transient perceptual distortions and may generate so-called "bad trips" reminiscent of psychotic states, several other drugs generate syndromes that more closely resemble schizophrenia. The most important of these are two widely abused stimulants, amphetamine and cocaine, and phencyclidine, commonly called PCP or "angel dust."

The paranoid delusions induced by amphetamine and its derivative methamphetamine are particularly well known. To generate this psychotic symptom, repeated large doses are generally necessary. Such a regimen commonly produces irritability and a growing suspiciousness that often culminates in severe paranoia similar to that seen in some schizophrenic patients.

Amphetamine-induced paranoid delusions are responsible for much of the violent criminal activity engaged in by people who abuse this drug. A virtually identical pattern is observed with repeated use of cocaine. Al-

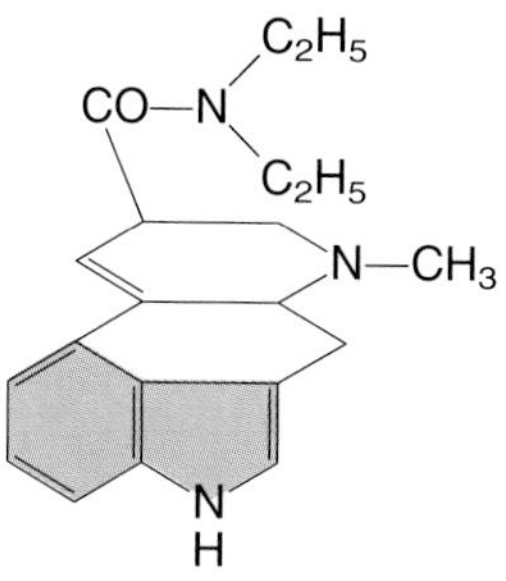

Lysergic acid diethylamide
(LSD)

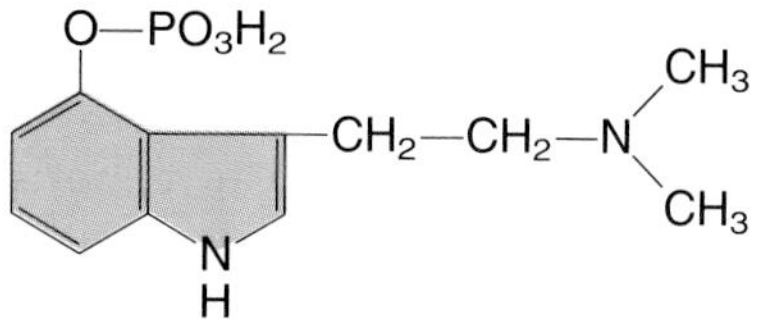

Psilocybin

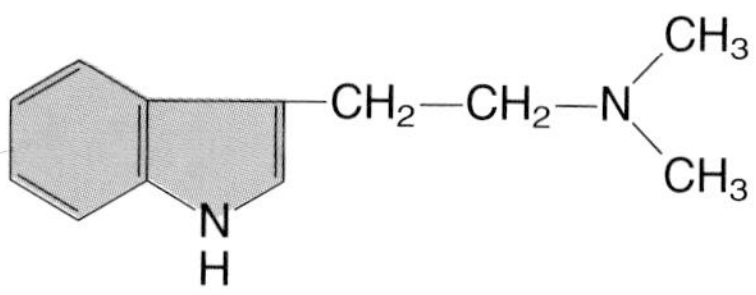

Dimethyltryptamine

Hallucinogens related to serotonin. Indole rings are highlighted by color.

Three drugs that can induce symptoms that mimic those observed in patients with schizophrenia.

Amphetamine

Cocaine

Phencyclidine (PCP)

though the paranoia recedes after withdrawal from the drug, once these symptoms appear it becomes increasingly likely that they will recur with subsequent stimulant use.

It has been argued that people who abuse stimulants manifest paranoid symptoms because they have a predisposition to psychotic behavior and that all the drugs are doing is activating a latent abnormality. There is evidence that this is actually true in some cases. For example, schizophrenic patients whose symptoms are in remission may have a flagrant recurrence after ingesting a small amount of amphetamine. Yet there is also persuasive evidence that stimulant abuse could make anyone psychotic. In studies done many years ago, in which repeated large doses of amphetamine were administered to normal volunteers under controlled conditions, every subject began to experience paranoid delusions within a week of beginning this regimen. Furthermore, recent studies of patients treated for cocaine dependency found that at least half had experienced both paranoid delusions and auditory hallucinations. The incidence of such reactions is particularly high when cocaine and methamphetamine are taken as "crack" and "ice" respectively, volatile forms whose effects closely resemble those of intravenous administration. Although it can be argued that drug abusers are not representative of the normal population, it is obvious that an enormous number of people are susceptible to the expression of psychotic behavior.

Like other psychoactive drugs, the stimulants have powerful effects on brain neurotransmitters (in this case, the catecholamines). Amphetamine has multiple actions—promoting the release of catecholamines, blocking their degradation by monoamine oxidase, and inhibiting their synaptic reuptake—all of which augment catecholaminergic neurotransmission. Cocaine's major effects are believed to be due primarily to increased synaptic action of dopamine as a result of inhibition of the dopamine transporter. The evidence that stimulants may cause psychotic symptoms by augmenting the actions of catecholamines fits with the potent antipsychotic effects of drugs that block dopamine receptors (e.g., chlorpromazine).

Behaviors characteristic of schizophrenia can also be induced by repeated administration of an entirely different type of drug, PCP. Developed in the 1950s as an anesthetic for animals, PCP initially seemed potentially useful for minor surgical procedures in humans as well, because it produced an indifference to the surgery without a total loss of consciousness. Clinical use of PCP was short-lived, however, because many patients experienced postoperative side effects, including agitation, paranoia, and hallucinations, that often lasted for days after treatment. Extensive psychological tests of normal volunteers under the influence of relatively small doses of PCP, which were not sufficient to cause anesthesia, revealed changes in their thought patterns that were characteristic of people with schizophrenia. Frequently, the volunteers also showed the social withdrawal and reduced emotional expression that is often displayed by schizophrenic patients.

PCP is no longer used clinically, but it is widely abused. It can be snorted or smoked, with rapid onset of effects, including the altered state of consciousness its users find so desirable. As with stimulant abuse, chronic use of PCP can lead to violent criminal behavior. Some abusers also develop characteristic movement abnormalities, like those seen in patients with catatonic-type schizophrenia.

PCP is of special interest because it influences the mind without exerting a primary effect on neurotransmission via brain monoamines. Instead, its target, at the relatively low nonanesthetic doses that induce psychosis, is a receptor for glutamate, which is the most abundant excitatory neurotransmitter in the brain. The particular glutamate receptor protein to which PCP binds is distinguished by its affinity for the synthetic amino acid agonist, N-methyl-D-aspartate (NMDA). This glutamate receptor also contains a gated Ca^{2+} channel.

The way in which PCP interacts with the NMDA receptor is worth some attention, because it illustrates just how unexpected drug actions

A computer-generated model of glutamate.

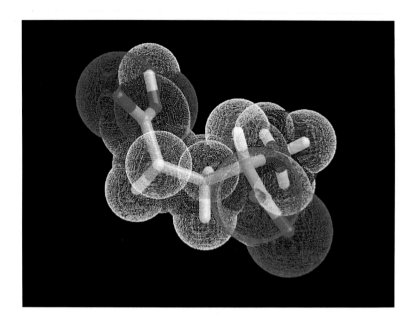

may be. Whereas glutamate induces ion-channel opening and entry of Ca^{2+} into the neuron by binding to a site on the outer surface of the receptor protein, PCP regulates ion-channel function via a binding site located within the channel itself. When PCP binds to this site, passage of Ca^{2+} through the channel is blocked. Because PCP acts at a binding site different from that of the receptor's natural ligand, it is called a noncompetitive inhibitor, meaning that high concentrations of glutamate (or NMDA) cannot compete with it by displacing it and overcoming its inhibitory effect.

The finding that psychotic reactions are produced by drugs with such different pharmacological spectra as PCP on the one hand and amphetamine and cocaine on the other supports the idea that different subtypes of schizophrenia may have different causes. The prominent paranoid symptoms elicited by amphetamine and cocaine are reminiscent of those seen in patients with paranoid-type schizophrenia. In contrast, PCP results in relatively more disordered thought and emotional withdrawal, as in patients with disorganized-type schizophrenia. Nevertheless, the great overlap among the various drug-induced forms of psychotic behavior, as well as among the various spontaneous forms, defies such neat distinctions, underscoring the difficulty we can expect to face in the search for the causes of this heterogeneous disorder.

Antipsychotic Drugs and Dopamine Receptors

In Chapter 5, we saw that certain effective antipsychotic agents were believed to work by blocking dopaminergic neurotransmission. For this reason, pharmaceutical companies interested in developing improved treatments for schizophrenia have concentrated on drugs that influence dopamine receptors, examining many relatives of chlorpromazine (called phenothiazines) as well as other types of compounds, such as haloperidol, a butyrophenone. The process of drug development was complicated by the discovery more than 20 years ago that there was more than one type of dopamine receptor.

The first clue that there were multiple dopamine receptors came from studies of dopamine-induced increases in the level of the second messenger cyclic AMP in fragments of brain tissue. As expected, chlorpromazine, which was known to be a dopamine receptor antagonist, blocked the effect of dopamine; but surprisingly, haloperidol, a very potent antipsychotic, did not share this effect. These apparently contradictory results stimulated extensive direct binding studies with a wide range of drugs used to treat schizophrenia. The upshot was that the drugs varied greatly in their rela-

Three Commonly Used Antipsychotic Drugs

	CLASS	MAJOR SIDE EFFECTS	ADVANTAGES
Fluphenazine	Phenothiazine	Movement disorders	Injected in time-release form
Haloperidol	Butyrophenone	Movement disorders	Few other side effects
Clozapine	"Atypical"	Reduces white blood cells, sometimes drastically	No movement disorders, improves negative symptoms

A computer-generated model of dopamine.

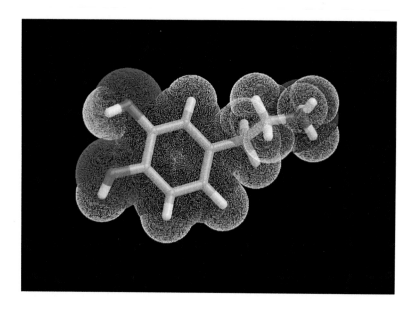

F

C=O

CH₂

CH₂

CH₂

N

OH

Cl

Haloperidol

tive binding to two different dopamine receptors, called D_1 and D_2. Haloperidol bound very well to D_2 but relatively poorly to D_1, whereas chlorpromazine bound fairly well to both D_1 and D_2. Attempts to correlate the clinical efficacy of these and many other drugs with their relative binding to D_1 or D_2 suggested that the antipsychotic effect was due to blockade of D_2 and that the effects on D_1 appeared irrelevant.

The discrepant effects of haloperidol and chlorpromazine on cyclic AMP levels in brain fragments were later explained by the finding that D_1 and D_2 each activate different types of G proteins. Dopamine binding to the D_1 receptor activates a G protein that leads to increased synthesis of cyclic AMP (by stimulating adenylate cyclase), whereas dopamine binding to the D_2 receptor activates a different G protein that actually reduces cyclic AMP levels (by inhibiting adenylate cyclase). Haloperidol's inability to bind the D_1 receptor explains its failure to block the dopamine-induced increase in cyclic AMP levels. Although chlorpromazine binds both D_1 and D_2 receptors, its net effect is to block dopamine's activation of D_1, thereby preventing elevation of cyclic AMP.

Drugs that inhibit D_2 receptors are very valuable, but they also produce troubling side effects, particularly strange and uncontrollable movements. In Chapter 5, we focused on the alarming appearance of acute Parkinsonian symptoms with administration of high doses of chlorpromazine. This phenomenon is now known to be due to inhibition of D_2 receptors, which are highly concentrated in the basal ganglia, brain structures that control many aspects of body movement. But movement abnormalities are also commonly observed even at much lower doses. One form, called akathisia, refers to jitteriness, sometimes verging on extreme excitement. Another form, akinesia, refers to a reduction in movement that may be accompanied by apathy and withdrawal. Patients who take these drugs for years may also develop a particularly serious form of movement disorder called tardive dyskinesia, which may become irreversible if the drug is not discontinued. A particularly distressing finding was that a drug's potency in inducing movement disorders was highly correlated with its potency in blocking D_2 receptors and so seemed to be inextricably related to its antipsychotic effects, which were also believed to be due to interaction with D_2.

This relationship between movement abnormalities and antipsychotic effect has been carefully examined in studies using the phenothiazine fluphenazine. Fluphenazine is widely used because it is available in an injectable form that is slowly released into the bloodstream, providing therapeutic levels for at least two weeks. This slow-release form is valuable for many schizophrenic patients who neglect to take antipsychotic medication in pill form.

Because intramuscular injection of fluphenazine gives rise to a fairly steady plasma drug level, detailed studies have been performed correlating plasma fluphenazine levels with antipsychotic effects and with disabling movement abnormalities. The results confirmed that the therapeutic effect could be achieved in some fortunate patients at a plasma level that did not produce disabling movement abnormalities; however, at the same plasma level, many other patients either had disabling side effects or showed no improvement, or both. Increasing the dose (and the plasma level) increased the antipsychotic effect but disproportionately increased the movement abnormalities. The upshot was that for many patients, the price of alleviating psychotic symptoms was a form of movement abnormality. This price accounts, in part, for the poor patient compliance and the frequent resort to sustained-release injections. The linkage of therapeutic and toxic effects appeared to be an insurmountable problem, since both antipsychotic activity and movement disorders seemed to be correlated with D_2 blockade.

Subsequently, this correlation was challenged by experience with another drug, clozapine, which is neither a phenothiazine nor a butyrophenone and is currently classified as "atypical." Clozapine was introduced

Fluphenazine

for the treatment of schizophrenia in 1969 by the Swiss pharmaceutical company Sandoz. Despite its antipsychotic effect, clozapine quickly fell out of favor when it was found to suppress markedly the white blood cell count of some patients, leading to several deaths from infection. Because of this disastrous side effect, U.S. approval was withheld, and the drug was used with extreme caution in Europe. Interest in clozapine was maintained because it did not produce movement disorders and so could be given to patients who found phenothiazines or butyrophenones intolerable.

Clozapine's ability to combat psychosis without producing movement disorders shattered what appeared to be an unbreakable coupling between

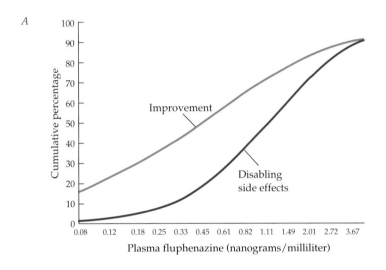

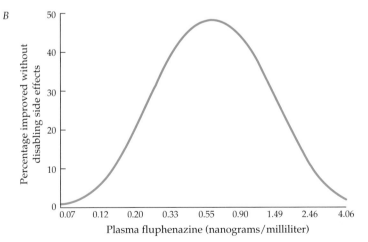

Graphs showing alleviation of symptoms and development of disabling side effects as a function of plasma levels of a slow-release form of fluphenazine that produces sustained blood levels when injected every two weeks. *(A)* Improvement and disabling side effects as a function of plasma fluphenazine. *(B)* Risk–benefit as a function of plasma fluphenazine.

Chapter 7

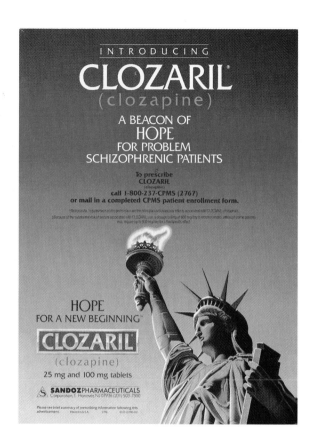

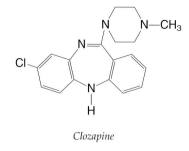

Clozapine

these two effects. Direct binding studies indicate that clozapine's association with D_2 receptors is relatively weak. This is consistent with the absence of abnormal movements; however, it also means that a drug can be an effective antipsychotic without producing substantial D_2 blockade. Might there be another type of dopamine receptor that clozapine binds in order to produce its antipsychotic effect?

Using variants of the techniques of cDNA cloning described in the previous chapters, investigators have recently discovered three new brain dopamine receptors, called D_3, D_4, and D_5. Furthermore, the evidence suggests that two of these dopamine receptor types exist in more than one form, and there are hints of still further diversity. The properties of D_3, D_4, and D_5 receptors had been obscured in previous binding studies by the greater prominence of D_1 and D_2 receptors, whose cDNAs have also been cloned. Each of these cDNAs has been introduced into suitable lines of

Relative binding of haloperidol and clozapine to D_2 receptors in the basal ganglia of the human brain measured by positron-emission tomography (PET). The three people whose brains were examined in this study each received raclopride, a drug that specifically binds the D_2 receptor. The raclopride was labeled with an isotope of carbon, [11C], that emits positrons, making it detectable by a scanner that measures these subatomic particles. Since the [11C] raclopride is concentrated in the basal ganglia, many positrons are emitted from this brain region. Their source is calculated by the scanner in computer-generated "slices" of regions of the brain, giving rise to a series of PET images. The person whose PET image is at the top takes no antipsychotic drugs, and thus had extensive binding of [11C] raclopride to D_2 receptors in the basal ganglia, as indicated by the red (most intense) and yellow (intense) isotope localization in that brain region. The person whose PET image is in the middle takes haloperidol, a potent D_2 ligand, which occupies the D_2 receptors in the basal ganglia so completely that there is virtually no binding of [11C] raclopride, as indicated by the blue color of the basal ganglia. The person whose PET image is at the bottom takes clozapine, which binds less well to the D_2 receptor than does haloperidol, and competes less well with [11C] raclopride, allowing enough to bind to emit a fairly intense yellow signal from the basal ganglia. Since doses of clozapine that effectively treat schizophrenia occupy only a limited number of D_2 receptors in the basal ganglia (as indicated by the availability of many receptors to bind [11C] raclopride), they do not produce the disabling movement disorders that are common with other antipsychotic drugs, such as haloperidol.

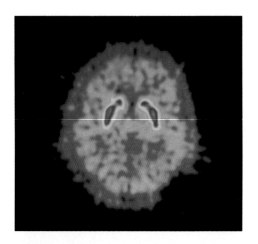
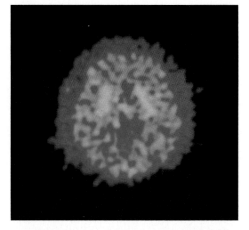
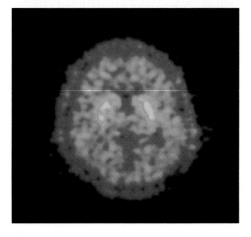

164   *Chapter 7*

human cells that are maintained in tissue culture, giving rise to cells that display one particular dopamine receptor on their surface and providing a basis for examining each receptor's binding affinity for a wide range of drugs.

Binding assays reveal that the D_4 receptor has a relatively high affinity for clozapine, suggesting that it, rather than the D_2 receptor, is the site of this drug's therapeutic action. Although the D_4 receptor is much scarcer in the brain overall than the D_2 receptor, it is relatively prominent in certain brain regions, such as the frontal cortex and the amygdala, which have been implicated in thought and emotion respectively. This raises the possibility that these brain regions may be specifically involved in schizophrenia. On the other hand, the D_4 receptor is relatively scarce in the basal ganglia, the structures that degenerate in Parkinson's disease and that are the major site of the D_2 receptors.

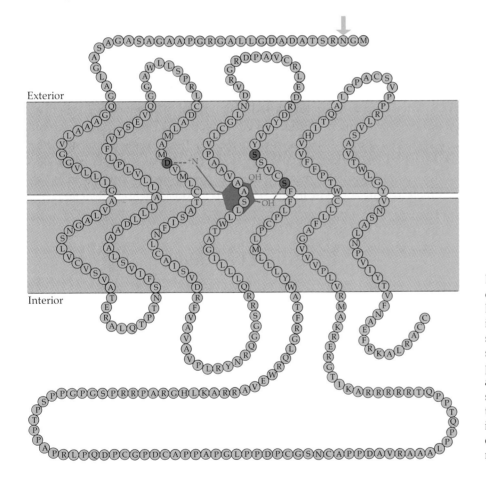

Diagram of the dopamine D4 receptor schematically depicting how it is believed to be situated in the plasma membrane, and showing the presumed binding site of dopamine (red), as proposed by Philip Seeman. Amino acids are represented by their standard single-letter abbreviations. A chain of sugars (arrow) is linked to an asparagine (N) on the extracellular part of the receptor.

The D_4 receptor has consequently become an important target for new drugs being developed to treat schizophrenia. It is hoped that it will prove possible to identify a D_4 antagonist that lacks clozapine's undesirable actions. What complicates matters is that clozapine also affects other dopamine receptors as well as certain serotonin receptors. It may be, therefore, that its distinctive therapeutic effect depends on interactions with the right mixture of receptors.

Besides not generating disabling movement disorders, clozapine has another great advantage, namely efficacy in a subset of schizophrenic patients whose symptoms are not alleviated by phenothiazines or butyrophenones. In these treatment-resistant patients so-called negative symptoms (e.g., social withdrawal, apathy, and emotional impoverishment) predominate over positive symptoms (e.g., paranoid delusions and hallucinations), which respond well to phenothiazines or butyrophenones. By alleviating negative symptoms, clozapine stimulates interest in social activities, which may aid greatly in rehabilitation.

Despite these advantages, clozapine is no magic bullet. It has the potentially lethal side effect of markedly reducing white blood cell levels in 1 to 2 percent of patients. To prevent this toxic effect, the white blood cell levels of all patients taking clozapine must be carefully monitored at frequent intervals; if these levels fall too far, administration of the drug should be discontinued. Furthermore, not all patients are responsive to the drug: most have only partial symptomatic relief, and some are troubled by side effects, such as drooling and sedation. Nevertheless, under controlled conditions and with the proper patients, clozapine has proven to be an extremely useful addition to the repertoire of antipsychotic drugs.

Future Directions

The current status of biological research on schizophrenia is quite similar to that of research on mood disorders. As with mood disorders, there is evidence that genes predispose to the development of schizophrenia, and it is expected that finding the genes responsible will improve our understanding of the disorder and point to new treatments. Again as with mood disorders, research on proteins that interact with neurotransmitters is valuable as a basis for the search for better therapeutic drugs.

Although these biological approaches offer the best hope for decisive advances in understanding and treatment, the terrible plight of people

DJW

by Dan E. Weisburd

David Jay Weisburd was born April 13, 1961, after sixteen hours of intense labor and a transverse presentation that the obstetrician tried to turn, with partial success. He was a very attractive infant, declared "perfect in every way" by the doting pediatrician who monitored David's growth and development. A walker at eleven months, a reader by the age of three, David showed an early love of numbers: while his nursery schoolmates ate paint and crayons and did finger smudges on butcher paper, David crammed pages full of numbers—up, down, and sideways. A gym coach at the Jewish Center said David seemed "unsure" of his body compared to other preschool children on the monkey bars.

Kindergarten was a huge disappointment for David, who began, nervously, to twist a tuft of hair, till he developed a bald spot many inches in diameter. Tested by a school psychologist, he was declared "a genius" and moved into a class for the highly gifted, where he could create his own structure and move at his own pace, which was rapid. He had a few loyal friends, plus a sister (two and a half years younger) whom he loved to taunt, and a brother (five years younger) whom he treasured and mentored. His sister and brother were also declared "gifted." At his departure from elementary school, David's sixth-grade teacher called him the brightest of all the highly gifted—"and painfully shy."

In junior high school he engaged in after-school sports, playing catcher, the most physical

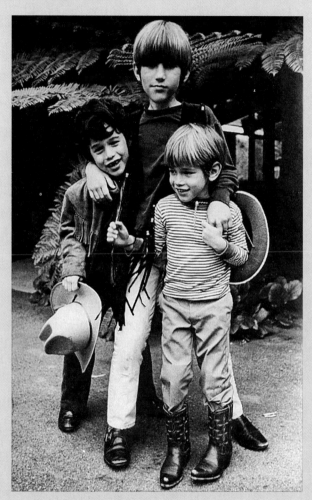

David Weisburd (*center*), about age 9, with his brother (*right*) and a cousin (*left*).

position, with a sense of abandon and disregard for the marvels that orthodontia had fashioned for him. Two nights a week he went to UCLA graduate school for classes in astronomy and cosmology, in which he predictably earned As. On weekends he tutored children who had difficulty in math and created a math fair for minority children in lower socioeconomic neighborhoods. Pro-social, active, grateful for his gifts and delighted to share them, David found life promising and exciting.

High school saw him become a long-distance runner and tennis player. When there was no teacher for calculus, he taught himself and tested perfectly in the Advanced Placement exam. Between eleventh and twelfth grade David attended Andover summer session, leading their tennis team to victory over Exeter while impressing his existential philosophy professor (who taught at Harvard) so much that he wrote a letter to us stating that David was the best student he had ever had, must go to Harvard, etc. David discovered sex at Andover, too, and pot. Confused by the philosophy and the intimacy, he relied more and more on marijuana throughout his senior year. While continuing to make his usual A grades, and scoring an almost perfect 1575 out of a possible 1600 on his SAT, he began showing some strange, uncharacteristic, volatile behaviors, including what may have been a drug-induced psychotic break at his senior prom.

Eligible to enter Harvard as a sophomore because of his many Advanced Placement achievements, David chose instead to enroll as a freshman because there were so many courses that interested him. He felt the calling to be "some kind of healer, who needed to know everything—perhaps a doctor of the mind, a psychiatrist." His grades were all outstanding, and when I visited him, at his invitation, for the Harvard–Yale game, I saw that he had made many male and female friends. I also found he had developed a disturbing set of attitudes, all of which seemed centered on the recreational use of drugs. My expressed concerns about Timothy Leary et al. were laughed off as "old fashioned."

With the encouragement of his Harvard adviser, David decided to take time off between his freshman and sophomore years "to explore the new age holistic practices that were out there" in northern California. It sounded treacherous to us, but David had always marched to his own beat, while we took bows for his uniqueness and his unorthodox ideas and accomplishments. So we supported the experiment, little knowing that he was coming apart. He got a degree in massage from one "institute," stood next to a vagrant who was stabbed through the heart in People's Park during a Berkeley uprising, burned out the engine of the VW van we had got him (which he then abandoned, selling it to a mechanic for a few hundred dollars to buy food), and was totally unprepared, as he stuffed a few wrinkled and dirty pieces of clothing into a tattered suitcase, to go back to Harvard. We were numb as we watched him board the plane that September.

Three weeks later he called. I remember hearing the hospital PA system in the background. "Don't worry, Dad, I can handle it. I've checked myself into the hospital. You won't believe this, but last night the entire football team, in the nude, chased me across Harvard Square and threw a grand piano at me. Now all the radio stations in the world are beaming their signals into my brain, saying the world wants me dead." His doctor got on the phone, said that David was much more ill than the Quincy House senior tutor could believe because of the smoke screen of David's brilliance, and urged us to come retrieve David as soon as possible and bring him to a psychiatric hospital nearer home. Two things were implied in what the doctor said: we were in for a long siege, and there was little or nothing that Harvard knew to do for this now less-than-perfect being whom they had so fervently courted only two years previously.

Because my wife and I were both moderately successful in our careers, and had substantial savings that we were willing to spend "to buy back his health," we naively set out to do just that in the private sector, falsely assuming that the "best" was out there and could make a difference. A couple of years and several savings accounts later, we were ready to try the public system (SSI, Medi-Cal, the works) because it couldn't be any worse than the conflicting, manipulative, high-cost nonsense that we had so far purchased in the name of hope.

David was refractory to all antipsychotic medications. He was zombied, made toxic, and, at times, incontinent. He was disruptive in day-treatment programs, a fire hazard in various residential settings, argumentative, even violent, and regularly kicked out of place after place, supposedly to preserve the "milieu" for others whose behavior was more "appropriate." The easy ones got the service, the sickest got the streets; that was what we saw time and again. On the outside David was jailed, robbed, lost in the Sierra foothills and in the Tenderloin of San Francisco, victim of an attempted rape. In and out of private, county, state, and university hospitals, he was diagnosed with everything in the *DSM-III*. Blood screens never showed he was still a

street-drug user. Frustrated doctors accused him of "cheeking the meds" because he did not respond as they felt he should to a particular dosage. He was a failure as a patient, obdurate. Doctor after doctor said "sorry" as David was dropped till, soon, he had been seen by dozens of psychiatrists, not to mention legions of interns and residents. At one particularly intriguing session, 30 doctors listened as David's case was presented and then voted on a diagnosis. But always the care that followed seemed to lead nowhere.

It was a nightmare in broad daylight. David was an enigma, one of those "dirty ones" walking down the street, disheveled and ranting at unseen assailants, a curiosity—even an object of fear. Lost, lonely, and full of terror, he tried to help himself in myriad desperate ways. He made a cave of his bedroom and lit candles everywhere. He danced an exotic ritual, eyes focused on the noonday sun. He tried acupuncture and sensory-deprivation tanks, mud baths and fasts. He stopped eating altogether, once, for days, convinced that if he ate the world would end, and so to save the world he was willing to starve. Nothing worked. His fall from what seemed a golden age appeared unstoppable, with little to hold on to except memories of the past achievements of a gifted youth sought after by prestigious universities and attractive and bright young women.

There were kindnesses, too, and competence, though not always, or not usually, from the most skilled and credentialed of caregivers. But more often than not there was the indignity of being treated like an object of derision and disgust as judges ordered him into locked treatment facilities that closely resembled the snakepits of another era. From somewhere he collected enough Seconals to make an attempt at suicide, only to have his stomach pumped in time with a solution of charcoal. And once, at 2 A.M., police officers showed compassionate restraint, putting aside their guns and nonviolently relieving him of an eight-inch butcher's knife, when terrifying paranoia had David convinced that someone was coming to kill him.

Trying to get the best and the latest for David, we prevailed upon a bright research psychiatrist to do 175 MRI (magnetic resonance imaging) "slices" of his brain, and to consult with a man from Aberdeen, Scotland, who was purportedly the best interpreter of those pictures. The conclusion of these two middle-aged men, after much ruminating over the artful shots of his frontal lobe, was that that sector of David's brain seemed to have shrunk ("just a tad") to about the size of their own, not what they'd expected in a man 20 years younger than themselves, which meant, perhaps . . . who knows what?

Many a valiant try has been made over the last 12 years to rescue this once-promising young man, who still, through it all, can show a momentary winning smile, a touch of grace and good manners, a fleeting hint of a whimsical sense of humor, and a gift for turning a meaningful phrase, if one can only wait out a lot of disconnectedness. Every once in a while now, David will put his arms around his mother or me and thank us for standing by him and being there through all these awful years. And we will reminisce about the good times, before the onset of his illness. His memory for past detail is keen, his thoughts insightful. But then, as we switch to something in the here and now, he gets lost and puzzled. His speech becomes aimless, rambling and polyclausal. He retains an incredibly expanded vocabulary, the product of hour-after-hour tours through one of his many dictionaries. But his communication skill rarely comes to any coherent conclusion, though it

with schizophrenia demands more immediate attention. Lulled by the promise of chlorpromazine and reserpine in the 1950s, we have prematurely dismantled a system for the humane treatment of those disabled by schizophrenia, and in so doing, we have caused many of them to be shamefully neglected.

When Adolf Wölfli, the artist whose colored drawing opens this chapter, was found to have delusions of persecution and auditory and visual hallucinations, he was hospitalized at the Waldau Asylum near Bern, Switzerland. He was 31 at the time and remained in the asylum until his death 35 years later. At the asylum he was sheltered, nourished, and protected from harm, the ward of a society which had no specific remedies to offer but was committed to caring for the mentally ill. Because he was frequently agitated and combative, he spent many years in relative isolation, mostly writing and drawing with crayons and pencil about himself as a supreme being, Saint Adolf, who ruled over a limitless world.

dazzles his fellow patients and more than an occasional therapist. They acknowledge his "brilliance," which pleases David very much.

David's third try on Clozaril [clozapine] has substantially reduced his "voices," and akathisia no longer has him frantically wearing out a pair of shoes a week. Sometimes David jokes about himself as an overstuffed human apothecary shop, but for the moment, thank goodness, he has been able to stop using the agents that bring on tardive dyskinesia.

As for the future, he still expresses a desire to go back to school to try again to do what he remembers doing so well—be a student. The age of computers came about while he lived more than a drugged decade as a psychiatric subject, and he shies away from giving them a try. At the moment he spends his days barefoot in smelly, dilapidated tennis shoes, sipping coffee and chain smoking with a friend, playing intricate improvised piano or guitar, and looking at faces in the shopping mall across from the board-and-care home where he lives with 30 other neurobiologically disabled persons. A lot of his rage seems to have subsided. Really, what he does mostly is wait. I wish better for him than what I realistically see in his immediate future. Perhaps when someone learns something more precise about the brain receptors involved, and someone else develops more appropriate medications to relieve the chemical chaos of it all, David's extraordinary mind will once again become an asset to him and not merely a perplexing composite of deficits for others to try to decode.

Dan E. Weisburd, a television writer and producer, is past-president of the California Alliance for the Mentally Ill (CAMI), an affiliate of the National Alliance for the Mentally Ill. He is currently editor and publisher of CAMI's quarterly publication, The Journal.

Although it would be naive to romanticize the conditions at the Waldau Asylum, they do represent a minimum standard of care that we must once again provide to those disabled with schizophrenia. Fortunately, a significant number of people afflicted with this disorder improve with the help of increasingly effective medications; and it is likely that Wölfli would have been among them. But so many others are neglected, and thousands languish homeless on our streets.

It is, of course, a great deal to ask of a society to care for several million people with this serious mental illness. The burden is especially great because many become ill in their teens or in early adulthood, are difficult to deal with, are sometimes violent and belligerent, and require care for many decades. Since the problem is so enormous, an increasing investment in a search for causes and cures is undoubtedly very cost-effective. But until those hopes are fulfilled, common decency demands a higher level of supervised care for these unfortunate people.

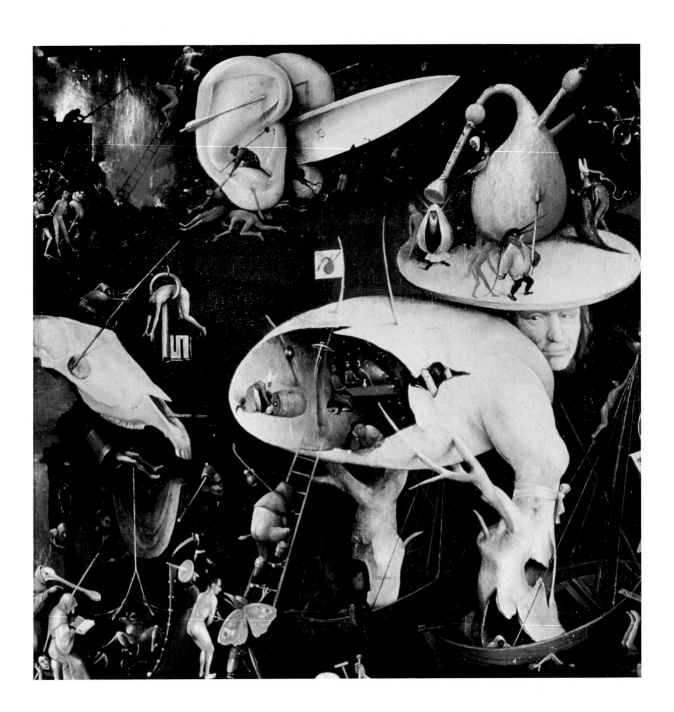

8

FEARS AND COMPULSIONS

In Chapters 6 and 7, we discussed disorders related to altered mood, on the one hand, and to suspiciousness and withdrawal, on the other. But the most common disorders that come to the attention of psychiatrists are related to yet another basic human trait, the tendency to be afraid. These conditions, collectively called the anxiety disorders, are characterized by irrational fears, often of savage intensity, and by specific behaviors that are designed to avoid these distressing feelings. In this chapter, we will explore the nature of the anxiety disorders and consider changing views of their cause and treatment.

Like all organisms, humans have evolved in an environment that is filled with danger. A major function of our nervous system is to evaluate situations for possible threats, and to find ways of avoiding or escaping

OPPOSITE: Detail from *Garden of Earthly Delights,* c. 1500, by Hieronymus Bosch.

them. One component of the nervous system, called the sympathetic nervous system, plays a critical role in such reactions. By releasing norepinephrine and epinephrine from nerve terminals and the adrenal glands, this specialized system activates receptors on vital organs, such as the heart, the blood vessels, and the sweat glands, thereby helping to mobilize the body for defense or escape (often called the "fight-or-flight" reaction).

The sympathetic nervous system is ultimately under the control of brain circuits that interpret evidence of danger. Although most indications of danger are learned from experience, the knowledge of some elaborate danger signals is actually inherited. For example, the Dutch ethologist Nickolaas Tinbergen found that chicks of certain species have an innate fear of silhouettes that resemble the shadows of their natural predators. Chicks

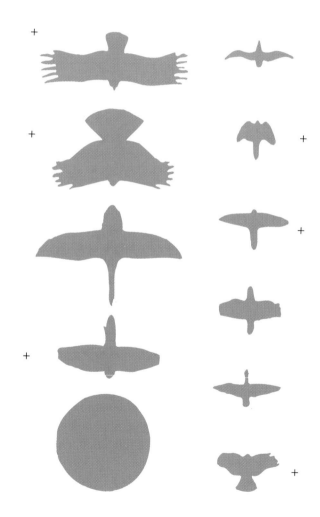

Silhouettes used to study innate alarm reactions in young birds. The shapes resembling shadows of birds' natural predators (+) elicited escape responses (crouching, crying, running for cover); silhouettes of innocuous species elicited no obvious response.

that were raised in isolation and had never seen hawks became agitated when exposed to shapes resembling hawks but did not react to the shapes of other, nonpredatory, birds. The chicks did not have to learn this response from experience: knowledge of the threatening shapes is genetically "hardwired" into their brains, along with the necessary connections to the neuronal circuits that control the fear response. A similar process of inheritance may underlie the innate fears that become exaggerated in certain human phobias, such as the fear of heights.

The higher brain centers not only call forth escape but also develop strategies for avoiding danger. Avoidance responses may involve transient mild activation of the sympathetic nervous system, sometimes called signal anxiety, which helps increase preparedness until it seems safe to relax. However, once the reliability of an avoidance reaction is established there may be no sympathetic activation. We cross at the green with equanimity.

An innate property of avoidance behavior, which can be demonstrated in humans as well as in animals, is that such behavior, once established, is difficult to erase. For example, if a mouse learns, through an appropriate training procedure, that a flash of light is occasionally followed by a painful shock, and that it can avoid the shock by pressing a button in response to the light, the mouse will continue to respond to the light signal long after the experimenter has permanently switched off the shock. This tendency to perpetuate avoidance behavior probably developed because species survive by erring on the side of caution. It is clearly more efficient for an organism to persevere in certain seemingly useless self-protective behaviors that cost it relatively little, rather than to risk omitting a particular action, only to find that, on a rare occasion, it prevents great pain. This natural tendency also plays a role in some of the inappropriate behaviors of people with anxiety disorders.

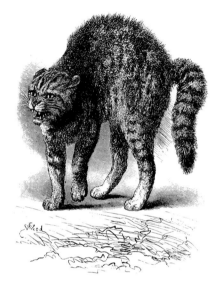

Cat prepared for "fight-or-flight." From Darwin's *The Expression of the Emotions in Man and Animals,* 1872.

Anxiety Disorders and the Concept of Neurosis

It is normal for humans to become anxious at times. What distinguishes people with anxiety disorders is that their behavior is not appropriate to the circumstances. For example, a soldier who becomes terrified on the battlefield is considered to be having a normal "fight-or-flight" reaction, whereas someone who experiences an unprovoked panic attack in a shopping mall is considered to be ill. But is it not possible that the second person is actually reacting normally to the shopping mall, in the light of his or her idiosyncratic experiences in such situations? The problem with this theory is that the patient will emphatically refute it, insisting that there is no good reason to be so afraid. Is it not possible, then, that the patient is simply unaware of the reasons?

The idea that anxiety disorders actually reflect unconscious mental processes was central to Sigmund Freud's development of psychoanalysis. Working from personal experience and the accounts of his patients, Freud concluded that humans are not conscious of many important learning experiences, especially sexual ones, partly because of their basis in infantile impressions that are not governed by adult thought processes. This unconscious learning may generate internal struggles that, in some people, result in what Freud called psychoneuroses (or neuroses).

If Freud's view is correct, however, why doesn't everyone have psychoneuroses? And of those who do, why do some have panic attacks, others (like Anna O. in Chapter 1) hysterical paralysis, and still others different neuroses entirely? Throughout his life, Freud struggled with the problem of how individuals chose a particular pattern of symptoms to cope with underlying conflicts. In the end, he would always fall back on the notion that "constitutional factors," presumably of genetic origin, were responsible. But he steadfastly maintained that these genetic tendencies expressed themselves through conflicts of unconscious mental forces—the essence of the neurotic process—that were ultimately understandable and treatable by psychological means.

In early editions of the *Diagnostic and Statistical Manual of Mental Disorders,* Freud's ideas gained formal recognition, and neurosis was established as a major diagnostic category. But in the third edition, *DSM-III,* published in 1980, this category was eliminated, a decision that reflected growing controversy about the usefulness of psychoanalytic ideas in the study and treatment of anxiety disorders. Since the term neurosis is still part of our general vocabulary, it is worthwhile to quote from the introduction of *DSM-III,* which explains why neurosis was eliminated as an official diagnostic entity:

> Throughout the development of *DSM-III* the omission of the *DSM-II* diagnostic class of Neuroses has been a matter of great concern to many clinicians, and requires an explanation. . . . Freud used the term both *descriptively* (to indicate a painful symptom in an individual with intact reality testing) and to indicate the *etiological process* (unconscious conflict arousing anxiety and leading to the maladaptive use of defense mechanisms that result in symptom formation). At the present time, however, there is no consensus in

our field as to how to define "neurosis." Some clinicians limit the term to its descriptive meaning whereas others also include the concept of a specific etiological process. To avoid ambiguity the term *neurotic disorder* should be used only descriptively. . . . The term *neurotic process,* on the other hand, should be used when the clinician wishes to indicate the concept of a specific etiological process involving the following sequence: unconscious conflicts between opposing wishes or between wishes and prohibitions, which causes unconscious perception of anticipated danger or dysphoria, which leads to use of defense mechanisms that result in either symptoms, personality disturbance, or both.

The term *neurotic disorder* thus refers to a mental disorder in which the predominant disturbance is a symptom or group of symptoms that is distressing to the individual and is recognized by him or her as unacceptable and alien . . . : reality testing is grossly intact; behavior does not actively violate gross social norms (although functioning may be markedly impaired); the disturbance is relatively enduring or recurrent without treatment and is not limited to a transitory reaction to stressors; and there is no demonstrable organic etiology or factor. . . . Thus, the term *neurotic disorder* is used in *DSM-III* without any implication of a special etiological process. . . .

In the 1987 revision of *DSM-III,* called *DSM-III-R,* even the term neurotic disorder was eliminated, presumably because of lingering connotations, and there was virtually no mention of the word neurosis. Only the atheoretical descriptive term anxiety disorder remained.

Characteristics and Prevalence of Anxiety Disorders

In the 1980s, as the conceptualization of the anxiety disorders was changing, a survey of their prevalence, called the Epidemiological Catchment Area Study, was conducted under the sponsorship of the National Institute of Mental Health (NIMH). Research teams interviewed a total of 20,000 people in five different regions of the United States, called catchment areas—Baltimore, Durham, Los Angeles, New Haven, and St. Louis— to determine if they met the criteria (which changed during the study as *DSM-III* was revised to *DSM-III-R*) for any of the formally defined anxiety disorders either at the time of the study or at some previous time. The researchers used accepted epidemiological techniques to sample people representative of the general population in each area. The data they accumulated made it possible to estimate the lifetime prevalence of anxiety disorders in the United States, expressed as the percentage of the population who would fulfill the formal criteria for any of these disorders at some time in their lives. The lifetime prevalence was remarkably high not only for the disabling anxiety disorders (panic disorder, agoraphobia, and obsessive-compulsive disorder) but also for those that are usually less severe (simple phobias, social phobia, and generalized anxiety disorder).

The most common and least disabling of the anxiety disorders examined in the NIMH study are the simple phobias. They are called "simple" not to minimize their importance but because in each case they involve a very clearly defined dreaded object (e.g., snakes or spiders) or situation (e.g., heights or closed spaces). Since so many of us have mild aversions to such things, the diagnosis is made only if a person's dread is so intense that it leads to total avoidance of the feared object or situation, or to overwhelming anxiety if it must be encountered. Even according to these stringent criteria, at least one in ten people (twice as many women as men) have a simple phobia. This widespread occurrence is not always obvious be-

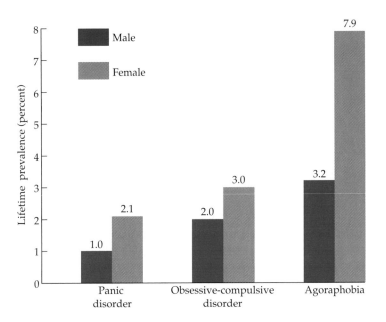

Lifetime prevalence of panic disorder, OCD, and agoraphobia as determined by the Epidemiological Catchment Area Study.

Chapter 8

cause most phobic people manage to avoid what they dread and think no more about it. If one lives in a modern urban setting, for example, a fear of snakes is hardly disabling.

The category of anxiety disorder called social phobia can be much more serious. It is formally defined in *DSM-III-R* as "a persistent fear of one or more situations in which the person is exposed to possible scrutiny by others and fears that he or she may do something or act in a way that will be humiliating or embarrassing." It affects men and women with equal frequency. The common experience of shyness and of a reluctance to make public speeches are not considered to be sufficiently abnormal to be included in this diagnostic category. But full-blown social phobia, which can become a great impediment to personal fulfillment and occupational success, was also found to be relatively common. That the lifetime prevalence of social phobia was about 3 percent came as a surprise, since relatively few people seek professional help for this condition.

The finding that more than 5 percent of people (somewhat more women than men) met the criteria for another descriptive category, called generalized anxiety disorder, was also unexpected. People in this category tend to have two types of problems: first, persistent and unrealistic worries about impending misfortunes; and second, multiple physical symptoms, including many that are attributable to hyperactivity of the sympathetic nervous system (e.g., rapid heart rate, palpitations, and excessive sweating). People with generalized anxiety disorder also tend to be tense, jittery, and easily fatigued. When they seek medical help, it is usually for physical complaints; thus, their underlying chronic anxiety is often overlooked.

The same cannot be said for panic disorder. Its symptoms include recurrent attacks of intense terror that come on without warning and without any apparent relationship to external circumstances. Although the attacks may last for only a few minutes, the experience is always excruciating. Terror triggers massive activation of the sympathetic nervous system, causing a wildly beating heart, sweating, and trembling. The distress can be so extreme that victims fear that they are dying or going crazy. Panic attacks may occur only once a week or even less frequently, but the victim's dread of a new episode may be virtually continual.

Panic disorder frequently coexists with an anxiety disorder called agoraphobia, which is a fear of public places (*agora* is Greek for marketplace) or of situations in which help might not be available. Both panic disorder and agoraphobia are twice as common in women as in men. In many cases, what the agoraphobic actually fears is the occurrence of a panic attack and the devastating feelings of vulnerability that would ensue if the attack hap-

Agoraphobia with Panic Attacks

The following case history from Nancy C. Andreasen's The Broken Brain *illustrates the progression from panic attacks to agoraphobia.*

Greg Miller is a 27-year-old unmarried computer programmer. When asked about his main problem, he replied, "I am afraid to leave my house or drive my car."

The patient's problems began approximately one year ago. At that time he was driving across the bridge that he must traverse every day in order to go to work. While driving in the midst of the whizzing six-lane traffic, he began to think (as he often did) about how awful it would be to have an accident on that bridge. His small, vulnerable VW convertible could be crumpled like an aluminum beer can, and he could die a bloody, painful death or, still worse, be crippled for life. His car could even hurtle over the side of the bridge and plunge into the river.

As he thought about these possibilities, he began to feel increasingly tense and anxious. He glanced back and forth at the cars on either side of him and became frightened that he might run into one of them. Then he experienced an overwhelming rush of fear and panic. His heart started pounding and he felt as if he were going to suffocate. He began to take deeper and deeper breaths, but this only increased his sense of suffocation. His chest felt tight and he wondered if he might be about to die of a heart attack. He certainly felt that something dreadful was going to happen to him quite soon. He stopped his car in the far right lane in order to try to regain control of his body and his feelings. Traffic piled up behind him with many honking horns, and drivers pulled around him yelling obscenities. On top of his terror, he experienced mortification. After about three minutes, the feeling of panic slowly subsided, and

pened in a public place. Some agoraphobics do not have full-blown panic attacks but nonetheless fear certain situations, such as being in a crowd or on a bus, in which they feel unprotected and exposed to some unidentified danger from which escape might be difficult. Often, agoraphobics can endure uncomfortable situations if they have a companion; however, in very severe cases, they are afraid to leave home, even if accompanied.

People with obsessive-compulsive disorder (OCD) display a very different pattern of disabling symptoms, combining recurrent unwelcome thoughts (obsessions) with repetitive behaviors designed to avoid a he was able to proceed across the bridge and go to work. During the remainder of the day, however, he worried constantly about whether or not he would be able to make the return trip home across the bridge without a recurrence of the same crippling fear.

He managed to do so that day, but during the next several weeks he would begin to experience anxiety as he approached the bridge, and on three or four occasions he had a recurrence of the crippling attack of panic. The panic attacks began to occur more frequently so that he had them daily. By this time he was overwhelmed with fear and began to stay home from work, calling in sick each day. He knew that his main symptom was an irrational fear of driving across the bridge, but he suspected that he might also have some type of heart problem. He saw his family doctor, who found no evidence of any serious medical illness, and who told him that his main problem was excessive anxiety. The physician prescribed a tranquilizer for him and told him to try to return to work.

For the next six months, Greg struggled with his fear of driving across the bridge. He was usually unsuccessful and continued to miss a great deal of work. Finally, he was put on disability for a few months and told by the company doctor to seek psychiatric treatment. Greg was reluctant and embarrassed to do this, and instead he stayed home most of the time, reading books, listening to records, playing chess on his Apple computer, and doing various "handyman" chores around the house. As long as he stayed home, he had few problems with anxiety or the dreadful attacks of panic. But when he tried to drive his car, even to the nearby shopping center, he would sometimes have panic attacks. Consequently, he found himself staying home nearly all the time and soon became essentially housebound.

Excerpt from *The Broken Brain*, Nancy C. Andreasen, copyright © 1984 by Nancy C. Andreasen. Reprinted by permission of HarperCollins, Publishers.

dreaded event (compulsions). The obsessions tend to be concerned with acts of aggression, such as losing control and harming someone, or with contamination, such as being infected with germs. Compulsive rituals are generally related to the obsessive thoughts. For example, repetitive washing is linked with obsessions about germs or dirt; compulsive checking may be associated with fear of harming someone. Failure to perform these compulsive acts properly may bring about intense anxiety, which is why this condition is classified with the anxiety disorders.

Freud, who was extremely interested in the symbolic content of obsessive-compulsive symptoms, taking them to be disguised manifestations of underlying conflicts, was struck by the victims' inability to free themselves of these symptoms:

> This is a mad disease, surely. I don't think the wildest psychiatric phantasy could have invented anything like it, and if we did not see it every day with our own eyes we could hardly bring ourselves to believe in it. Now do not imagine that you can do anything for such a patient by advising him to distract himself, to pay no attention to these silly ideas, and to do something sensible instead of his nonsensical practices. This is what he would like himself; for he is perfectly aware of his condition, he shares your opinion about his obsessional symptoms, he even volunteers it quite readily. Only he simply cannot help himself; the actions performed in an obsessional condition are supported by a kind of energy which probably has no counterpart in normal mental life.

Obsessive-compulsive disorder affects women somewhat more frequently than men; it may begin in childhood or early adulthood and tends to persist thereafter. Its severity and course are quite variable. Samuel Johnson, the famous eighteenth-century writer and lexicographer, seems to have suffered from a relatively mild form of OCD, at least according to contemporary accounts. His friend James Boswell recorded a number of "superstitious habits" that have the earmarks of compulsive rituals:

> He had another particularly, of which none of his friends ever ventured to ask an explanation. It appeared to me some superstitious habit, which he had contracted early, and from which he had never called upon his reason to disentangle him. This was his anxious care to go out or in at a door or passage by a certain number of steps from a certain point, or at least so as that either his right or his left foot, (I am not certain which,) should constantly make the first actual movement when he came close to the door or passage. Thus I conjecture: for I have, upon innumerable occasions, observed him suddenly stop, and then seem to count his steps with a deep earnestness; and when he had neglected or gone wrong in this sort or magical movement, I have seen him go back again, put himself in a proper posture to begin the ceremony, and, having gone through it, break from his abstraction, walk briskly on, and join his companion. . . . it is requisite to mention, that while talking or even musing as he sat in his chair, he commonly held his head to one side towards his right shoulder, and shook it in a tremendous manner, moving his body backwards and forwards, and rubbing his left knee in the same direction, with the

palm of his hand. In the intervals of articulating he made various sounds with his mouth, sometimes as if ruminating, or what is called chewing the cud, sometimes giving a half whistle, sometimes making his tongue play backwards from the roof of his mouth, as if clucking like a hen, and sometimes protruding it against his upper gums in front as if pronouncing quickly under his breath, *too, too, too:* all this accompanied sometimes with a thoughtful look, but more frequently with a smile.

Johnson's symptoms were clearly not disabling and had no obvious effect on his literary productivity. The case of the billionaire businessman and philanthropist Howard Hughes falls at the other extreme. Hughes was preoccupied with a fear of germs, which he combated with elaborate and bizarre grooming rituals. His well-known deterioration to a disheveled recluse poignantly demonstrates how devastating this type of anxiety disorder may be.

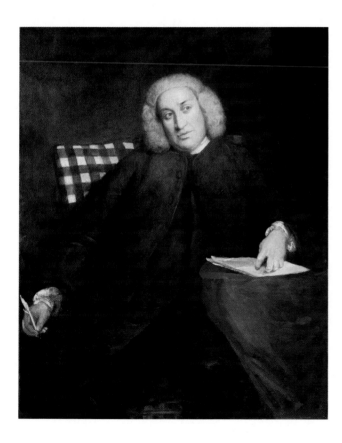
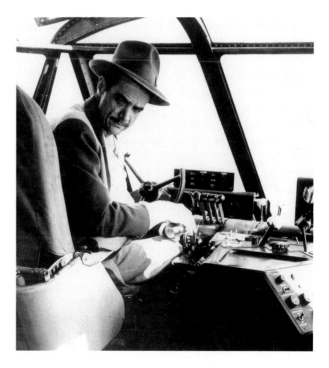

Samuel Johnson *(left)* and Howard Hughes, who had markedly different forms of obsessive-compulsive disorder.

An OCD Attack

The patient, a psychologist with obsessive-compulsive disorder, describes his illness. (Excerpted from Judith L. Rapoport's The Boy Who Couldn't Stop Washing.)

I'm driving down the highway doing 55 miles per hour. I'm on my way to take a final exam. My seat belt is buckled and I'm vigilantly following all the rules of the road. No one is on the highway—not a living soul.

Out of nowhere an obsessive-compulsive disorder (OCD) attack strikes. It's almost magical the way it distorts my perception of reality. While in reality no one is on the road, I'm intruded with the heinous thought that I *might* have hit someone . . . a human being! God knows where such a fantasy comes from.

I think about this for a second and then say to myself, "That's ridiculous. I didn't hit anybody." Nonetheless, a gnawing anxiety is born. An anxiety I will ultimately not be able to put away until an enormous emotional price has been paid.

I try to make reality chase away this fantasy. I reason, "Well, if I hit someone while driving, I would have *felt* it." This brief trip into reality helps the pain dissipate . . . but only for a second. Why? Because the gnawing anxiety that I really did commit the illusionary accident is growing larger—so is the pain.

The pain is a terrible guilt that I have committed an unthinkable, negligent act. At one level, I know this is ridiculous, but there's a terrible pain in my stomach telling me something quite different.

Again, I try putting to rest this insane thought and that ugly feeling of guilt. "Come on," I think to myself, "this is *really* insane!"

But the awful feeling persists. The anxious pain says to me, *"You really did hit someone."* The attack is now in full control. Reality no longer has meaning. My sensory system is distorted. I have to get rid of the pain. Checking out this fantasy is the only way I know how.

I start ruminating, "Maybe I did hit someone and didn't realize it . . . oh my God! I might have killed somebody! I have to go back and check." Checking is the only way to calm the anxiety. It brings me closer to truth somehow. I can't live with the thought that I actually may have killed someone—I have to check it out.

Now I'm sweating . . . literally. I pray this outrageous act of negligence never happened. My fantasies run wild. I desperately hope the jury will be merciful. I'm particularly concerned about whether my parents will be understanding. After all, I'm now a criminal. I must control the anxiety by checking it out. Did it really happen? There's always an infinitesimally small kernel of truth (or potential truth) in all my OC fantasies.

I think to myself, "Rush to check it out. Get rid of the hurt by checking it out. Hurry back to check it out. God, I'll be late for my final exam if I check it out. But I have no choice. Someone could be lying on the road, bloody, close to death." Fantasy is now my only reality. So is my pain.

I've driven five miles farther down the road since the attack's onset. I turn the car around and head back to the scene of the mythical mishap. I return to the spot on the road where I "think" it "might" have occurred. Naturally, nothing is there. No police car and no bloodied body. Relieved, I turn around again to get to my exam on time.

Feeling better, I drive for about 20 seconds and then the lingering thoughts and pain start gnawing away again. Only this time they're even more intense. I think, "Maybe I should have pulled *off* the road and checked the side brush where the injured body was thrown and now lies? Maybe I didn't go *far enough* back on the road and the accident occurred a mile farther back."

The pain of my possibly having hurt someone is now so intense that I have no choice—I really see it this way.

I turn the car around a second time and head an extra mile farther down the road to find the corpse. I drive by quickly. Assured that this time I've gone far enough I head back to school to take my exam. But I'm not through yet.

"My God," my attack relentlessly continues, "I didn't get *out* of the car to actually *look* on the side of the road!"

So I turn back a third time. I drive to the part of the highway where I think the accident happened. I park the car on the highway's shoulder. I get out and begin rummaging around in the brush. A police car comes up. I feel like I'm going out of my mind.

The policeman, seeing me thrash through the brush, asks, "What are you doing? Maybe I can help you?"

Well, I'm in a dilemma. I can't say, "Officer, please don't worry. You see, I've got obsessive-compulsive disorder, along with 4 million other Americans. I'm simply acting out a compulsion with obsessive qualities." I can't even say, "I'm really sick. Please help me." The disease is so insidious and embarrassing that it cannot be admitted to anyone. Anyway, so few really understand it, including myself.

So I tell the officer I was nervous about my exam and pulled off to the roadside to throw up. The policeman gives me a sincere and knowing smile and wishes me well.

But I start thinking again. "Maybe an accident did happen and the body has been cleared off the road. The policeman's here to see if I came back to the scene of the crime. God, maybe I really did hit someone . . . why else would a police car be in the area?" Then I realize he would have asked me about it. But would he, if he was trying to catch me?

I'm so caught up in the anxiety and these awful thoughts that I momentarily forget why I am standing on the side of the road. I'm back on the road again. The anxiety is peaking. Maybe the policeman didn't know about the accident? I should go back and conduct my search more *thoroughly*.

I want to go back and check more . . . but I can't. You see, the police car is tailing me on the highway. I'm now close to hysteria because I honestly believe someone is lying in the brush bleeding to death. Yes . . . the pain makes me believe this. "After all," I reason, "why would the pain be there in the first place?"

I arrive at school late for the exam. I have trouble taking the exam because I can't stop obsessing on the fantasy. The thoughts of the mystical accident keep intruding. Somehow I get through it.

The moment I get out of the exam I'm back on the road checking again. But now I'm checking two things. First that I didn't kill or maim someone and second, that the policeman doesn't catch me checking. After all, if I should be spotted on the roadside rummaging around the brush a second time, how in the world can I possibly explain such an incriminating and aimless action? I'm totally exhausted, but that awful anxiety keeps me checking, though a part of my psyche keeps telling me that this checking behavior is ridiculous, that it serves absolutely no purpose. But, with OCD, there is no other way.

Finally, after repeated checks, I'm able to break the ritual. I head home, dead tired. I know that if I can sleep it off, I'll feel better.

Sometimes the pain dissipates through an escape into sleep.

I manage to lie down on my bed—hoping for sleep. But the incident has not totally left me—nor has the anxiety. I think, "If I really did hit someone, there would be a dent in the car's fender."

What I now do is no mystery to anyone. I haul myself up from bed and run out to the garage to check the fenders on the car. First I check the front two fenders, see no damage, and head back to bed. But . . . *did I check it well enough?*

I get up from bed again and now find myself checking the *whole body* of the car. I know this is absurd, but I can't help myself. Finally . . . finally, I disengage and head off to my room to sleep. Before I nod off, my last thought is, "I wonder what I'll check next?"

Excerpt from *The Boy Who Couldn't Stop Washing*, Judith L. Rapoport, copyright © 1989 by New American Library. Reprinted by permission of Penguin U.S.A.

Genetic Predisposition

Because for many years anxiety disorders were considered to be mostly due to psychological factors, little attention was paid to observations that they tend to run in families. Recently, however, with the growth of interest in the role of biological factors in mental illness, this state of affairs has begun to change. Researchers are now accumulating considerable evidence suggesting that specific anxiety disorders depend on an underlying genetic predisposition. For example, several family studies currently under way indicate that first-degree relatives of patients with panic disorder are at substantially greater risk for this condition than members of the general population.

Although these family studies of panic disorder are not nearly so extensive as those of mood disorders or schizophrenia, they are supported by a number of animal studies. Particularly noteworthy is the case of Alleghany Sue, a champion pointer who became exceptionally fearful after a normal early life as a hunting dog. Inbreeding of her descendants has produced a strain of dogs that behave normally as puppies but begin to manifest intense anxiety in adolescence or early adulthood, the same developmental periods in which panic attacks often begin in people. Like panic attacks in many people, the dogs' extreme fearfulness is situation-dependent. Two consistent triggers of panic in these dogs are presentation of novel situations and exposure to humans. In the absence of these provocative stimuli, the dogs behave normally; they show no symptoms when interacting with other dogs.

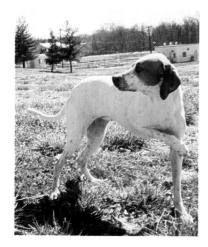

Alleghany Sue.

Dogs are not alone in displaying a hereditary propensity to fearfulness. In Chapter 2 we saw that mice can be bred for fearful behavior and that more than one gene interacts to give rise to this so-called emotionality. The availability of these animal models of inherited tendencies to fearfulness could be extremely helpful in the search for the genes that control anxiety in humans, since these genes could prove to be the same in all species.

There is also growing evidence for a genetic predisposition to OCD. Some of this evidence is anecdotal. The patient who was obsessed with the fear that he might have hit someone with his car (his story appears in a box on previous pages) writes:

> My son Jeffrey, age five, has had the illness since at least age two. My two brothers most probably have the disease, though less severely. There is a good chance my nephew, age eight, has OCD as well as my father and his father also. I can write this here, but families with OCD almost never tell each other about it if they can help it.

A particularly interesting lead in the search for a genetic basis for OCD comes from recent evidence that, in some families, it may be an alternative or additional expression of a genetic disorder of children and adults called Gilles de la Tourette syndrome, or Tourette's disorder. The pattern of transmission of Tourette's disorder, which affects about one person in 2000, is consistent with autosomal dominant inheritance. Patients with Tourette's disorder display peculiar involuntary behaviors called tics, which may include uncontrollable shouting or mumbling of obscene words as well as involuntary nodding, sniffing, hopping, and protrusion of the tongue (reminiscent of some of Samuel Johnson's symptoms). Many first-degree relatives of such patients have more limited tics, suggesting that the gene is variably expressed. In certain families with Tourette's disorder there is also a high incidence of OCD. Since in such families many of those affected with OCD are female, whereas their relatives with Tourette's disorder are largely males, the possibility of sex-influenced inheritance is raised.

Support for a relationship between these disorders comes not only from studies of families first identified because of Tourette's disorder but also from studies of families first identified because of OCD. Some of these OCD families have a much higher incidence of Tourette's disorder and tics than the general population; however, this is not true of all OCD families. This finding suggests that OCD, which is so much more common than Tourette's disorder, is genetically heterogeneous.

Drugs That Affect Catecholamine Receptors

Since fear is always accompanied by activation of the sympathetic nervous system and release of catecholamines, it would seem reasonable to expect that drugs that block these processes would be useful in treating anxiety disorders. Such an expectation would be heightened by the acceptance of a classical theory about the experience of fear formulated at the turn of the century by the American psychologist William James and the Danish physiologist Carl Lange. James and Lange believed that physiological responses, such as a rapid heartbeat, are a cause rather than a result of experiencing fear and that it is our awareness of physiological cues that is critical to our feeling afraid.

Were the James-Lange theory correct, fear could be mitigated by blocking the receptors that are activated by sympathetic nervous system discharge. In fact, there is some evidence that just such a simple remedy can be effective in people with performance anxiety, a limited form of social phobia that is not usually severe enough to warrant this formal diagnosis. Sufferers become fearful immediately before and during public performances such as making a speech, playing music, or competing in a sport. For example, a great many professional musicians report some degree of recurrent stage fright; among them have been such outstanding artists as pianist Artur Rubinstein and cellist Pablo Casals.

Performance anxiety has been successfully treated with drugs like propranolol, an antagonist of the beta-adrenergic receptor (i.e., a beta-blocker). When activated by norepinephrine, beta-adrenergic receptors,

Propanolol

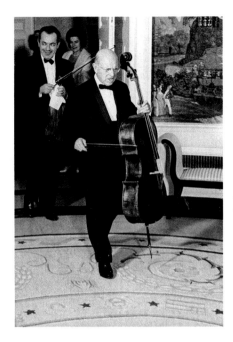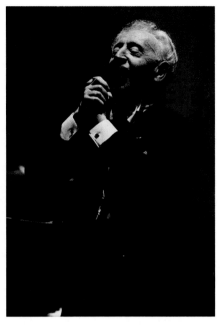

Pablo Casals *(left)* and Artur Rubinstein, who suffered from performance anxiety.

which are concentrated in several organs, including the heart, can so increase the heart rate that a performer becomes acutely aware of a heaving chest and a throbbing pulse. Perception of these symptoms elicits yet more anxiety and further activation of the sympathetic nervous system. A beta-blocker that attenuates these peripheral manifestations of anxiety in effect interrupts a positive feedback mechanism. Performers may find beta-blockers particularly attractive because they act primarily on the body rather than the brain and thus do not alter brain functions that could influence complex intellectual or artistic behavior. In sharp contrast, benzodiazepines (to be discussed shortly) alleviate anxiety by inhibiting brain processes and may therefore impair artistic performance.

Given the importance of catecholamines in mediating anxiety, it is very surprising that one of the most effective drugs against panic attacks is imipramine. This drug, already discussed in Chapters 5 and 6 because of its use as an antidepressant, is known to block neuronal reuptake of catecholamines and to augment their action as neurotransmitters. For this reason, imipramine might be expected to increase anxiety; yet, with sustained administration, it has actually proven to be valuable in preventing recurring panic attacks. What is more, monoamine oxidase inhibitors, another class of antidepressants that augment catecholamine effects, prevent panic attacks as well. Presumably, the adaptive brain changes produced after weeks of treatment with imipramine or monoamine oxidase inhibitors are responsible for their therapeutic efficacy against panic as well as depression. Nonetheless, how these drugs can alleviate two such disparate conditions remains, for the present, a mystery.

Benzodiazepines and GABA Receptors

The compounds most widely used for the management of anxiety are the benzodiazepines. Of these, diazepam (Valium) is probably the best known and alprazolam (Xanax) the most commonly prescribed for panic disorder. Both are descendants of chlordiazepoxide (Librium), whose antianxiety effects were discovered in the course of a routine screen of the influence of a wide range of chemicals on animal behavior conducted in the late 1950s. At that time, there was no reason to suspect that benzodiazepines would affect specific neurotransmitter receptors or, for that matter, influence the brain in any way. The story of these drugs is yet another reminder of the importance of chance observations in the identification of new classes of psychopharmacological agents.

We now know that the benzodiazepines exert their effect by binding to regulatory sites on receptors for gamma-aminobutyric acid (GABA). This amino acid is an inhibitory neurotransmitter that binds to receptors on a variety of brain neurons, including, presumably, some that are involved in circuits critical to the experience of anxiety. By augmenting GABA's inhibitory effect, benzodiazepines further turn down the activity of these neurons, thereby helping to reduce this uncomfortable feeling. Because GABA is so widely distributed, however (it is released as a neurotransmitter at about 40 percent of all brain synapses), it has been difficult to identify the critical locations in the brain where these antianxiety actions occur.

Given the extensive utilization of GABA, it should not be surprising that many types of GABA receptors have evolved. The vast majority, collectively called $GABA_A$ receptors, are targets of the benzodiazepines. This receptor class is structurally related to the nicotinic acetylcholine receptor: both are pentameric (composed of five separate subunits), and both are ligand-gated ion channels. But whereas the nicotinic acetylcholine receptor controls the passage of positive sodium ions, which depolarize the postsynaptic membrane and cause excitation, the $GABA_A$ receptor controls the

Diazepam

Alprazolam

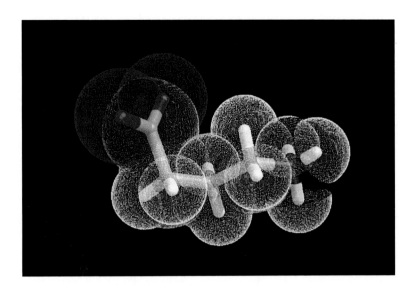

A computer-generated model of GABA.

passage of negative chloride ions, which hyperpolarize the postsynaptic membrane and cause inhibition.

Benzodiazepines bind to binding sites that reside on subunits of the $GABA_A$ receptor that are distinct from the subunits to which GABA itself binds. The binding of the benzodiazepines used in the treatment of anxiety, such as diazepam, to the benzodiazepine binding site favors a conformation of the pentameric $GABA_A$ receptor that enhances the interaction of GABA with its own binding site. Enhanced GABA binding increases chloride ion flow and postsynaptic inhibition, which presumably is responsible for the antianxiety effect. Because they bind to the benzodiazepine binding site in such a way as to augment GABA effects, diazepam and related drugs are classified as agonists of the benzodiazepine binding site.

To complicate matters, other related chemical compounds that also bind to the benzodiazepine binding site have different effects. For example, the binding of the experimental drug FG-7142 to the benzodiazepine binding site favors a different conformation of the $GABA_A$ receptor, resulting in diminished rather than enhanced binding of GABA to its binding site and thereby reducing GABA's inhibitory effect. Because its effect is inverse to that of diazepam, FG-7142 is classified as an inverse agonist of the benzodiazepine binding site. Yet another experimental drug, RO-15-1788, binds to the same site as diazepam and FG-7142 but neither enhances nor diminishes GABA's binding to its binding site. Since RO-15-1788

Interaction of GABA and a benzodiazepine with different subunits
of a GABA receptor. GABA binding changes the shape of the receptor, allowing Cl⁻ to flow into
the cell. Benzodiazepine binding
changes the properties of the receptor so that GABA binding is
enhanced. Although the diagram
shows sequential binding to illustrate this point, binding can actually occur in any order.

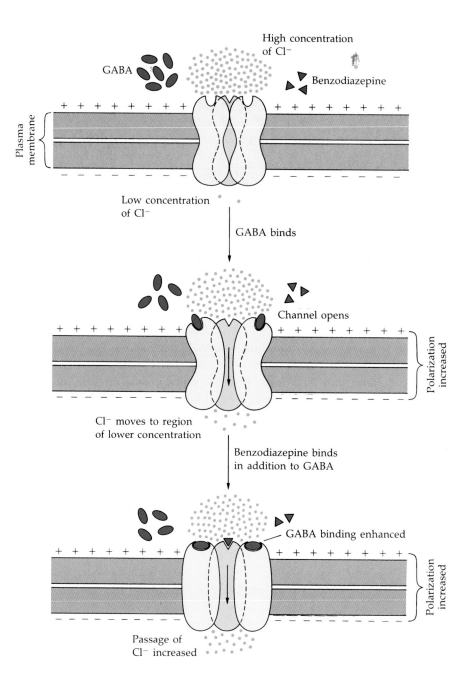

Chapter 8

blocks the binding of agonists such as diazepam, it is classified as an antagonist of the benzodiazepine binding site.

Identification of the $GABA_A$ receptor as the site of action of potent antianxiety drugs has raised the possibility that the brain normally modulates anxiety by making and releasing natural ligands for the benzodiazepine binding site. The search for natural ligands for opiate receptors, which led to the discovery of endorphins and enkephalins, was motivated by precisely the same reasoning. There is, in fact, considerable evidence that the brain contains an inverse agonist, a large peptide called diazepam binding inhibitor, that may play a role in promoting anxiety. The behavioral significance of this inverse agonist is presently being studied. In addition, the search continues for an endogenous agonist of the benzodiazepine binding site that might control anxiety.

To complicate matters further, there is extensive evidence indicating that numerous distinct varieties of $GABA_A$ receptors exist. Many different protein subunits that belong to this receptor family have been identified. Several research groups, including those of Eric Barnard in London and Peter Seeburg in Heidelberg, have succeeded in cloning cDNAs encoding many of these subunits. So far, they have found 13 unique protein subunits that can combine to form pentameric variants of the $GABA_A$ receptor.

In view of GABA's neurotransmitter activity at a vast number of brain synapses, it seems likely that different receptor subtypes evolved so that this single amino acid can exert a variety of physiological effects. This inference is supported by evidence (based on selective hybridization of the cDNAs for particular receptor subunits to specific brain regions) that certain forms of $GABA_A$ receptors are concentrated in unique populations of neurons, where they presumably play specialized roles and may interact in different ways with benzodiazepines. This evidence has implications for improved drug design: it may be that only certain subpopulations of $GABA_A$ receptors modulate anxiety, and drugs specific for these subpopulations could be more effective while causing fewer side effects. By transferring cloned cDNAs for different $GABA_A$ receptor subunits into appropriate cultured mammalian cells, researchers are creating particular $GABA_A$ receptors composed of specified subunit mixtures, which then can be evaluated as potential drug targets.

$GABA_A$ receptors are also of great interest because they are the site of action of barbiturates and alcohol, two other types of drugs that also alleviate anxiety by increasing GABA's inhibitory effect. The barbiturates, which were commonly used to treat anxiety before the discovery of the far greater efficacy of benzodiazepines, also augment GABA's effect by binding to and altering $GABA_A$ receptors; however, they do not bind to the same sites as

Phenobarbital

_Ethanol
(alcohol)_

the benzodiazepines. The oldest antianxiety drug, alcohol, also apparently works by augmenting the GABA-mediated flow of chloride ions, and there is growing evidence that a particular type of $GABA_A$ receptor subunit is alcohol's specific target. Given the enormous medical and social importance of alcohol, it is not surprising that the nature of its interactions with $GABA_A$ receptors is under active investigation.

In addition to their antianxiety effects, alcohol, barbiturates and benzodiazepines share yet another property: ingestion of any of these drugs in sufficient quantities and over sufficient periods leads to complex changes known as tolerance and physical dependence. Tolerance manifests itself as the need for progressively larger doses to produce the effect originally elicited by a smaller dose. Physical dependence is indicated by the appearance of withdrawal symptoms, such as anxiety and irritability, when administration of the drug is abruptly stopped. Withdrawal symptoms arise because, as discussed in Chapter 5, the nervous system uses many mechanisms to compensate for the sustained effects of drugs. In the case of alcohol, a barbiturate, or a benzodiazepine, the sustained effect is increased GABA-mediated inhibition, which provokes compensatory changes that favor activation. When the drug is withdrawn, these compensatory mechanisms are unopposed, leading to hyperactivity of the previously inhibited neurons.

In practice, most patients treated with benzodiazepines for anxiety disorders do not manifest substantial tolerance or physical dependence unless they are given large doses. But the enormous prevalence of alcoholism has intensified interest in compensatory changes in $GABA_A$ receptors.

Drugs for Obsessive-Compulsive Disorder

Although patients with obsessive-compulsive disorder experience considerable anxiety, they get little or no relief from benzodiazepines. Surprisingly, both obsessive and compulsive behavior can be significantly diminished by certain drugs that were originally developed as antidepressants.

By now, it should come as no surprise that the discovery of the value of antidepressants in the treatment of OCD sprang from an accidental observation. In 1969, the Spanish psychiatrist J. J. Lopez-Ibor found that obsessional symptoms of depressed patients were alleviated by intravenous injections of clomipramine, a relative of imipramine that was widely used as an antidepressent in Europe. This finding led to controlled clinical trials that established clomipramine's value as therapy for OCD.

In the course of these studies, it was observed that the value of antidepressants in the treatment of OCD appeared to be correlated with their potency as inhibitors of the neuronal reuptake of serotonin rather than norepinephrine. Of the relatives of imipramine, clomipramine binds particularly well to the serotonin transporter and alleviates OCD. In contrast, another relative, desipramine, which blocks reuptake of norepinephrine but not of serotonin, has no value in the treatment of this disorder. The direct connection between inhibition of the serotonin transporter and symptom reduction is supported by the finding that fluoxetine, fluvoxamine, and sertraline, newer antidepressants that selectively block serotonin reuptake, are also effective in patients with OCD.

The discovery that obsessive-compulsive disorder responds to clomipramine has led to successful treatment of other patterns of uncontrollable behavior, such as trichotillomania (an irresistible impulse to pull out one's own hair) and onychophagia (compulsive nail biting). Clomipramine somewhat ameliorates both these conditions. Interestingly, it also helps control a similar self-mutilating behavior called canine acral lick, which afflicts Great Danes and German Shepherds; in this condition, paw licking is so excessive that the skin becomes ulcerated. The shared pharmacological responsivity suggests that all these apparently uncontrollable behaviors—human and nonhuman—have something in common, but the mechanism is at present unclear.

$$CH_2CH_2CH_2N(CH_3)_2$$

Clomipramine

Psychotherapy

More than any other of the serious conditions addressed by psychiatry, the anxiety disorders lend themselves to the wide range of psychological treatments collectively called psychotherapy. The major reason why this is so is that people with anxiety disorders hate their symptoms, know they need help, and are willing to talk about it. This is not always the case with the disorders we discussed in previous chapters: most manics claim to be persuaded of their transcendent excellence, depressives of their worthlessness, and schizophrenics of the malevolence of those they believe are plotting against them or controlling their minds. Such patients are, in general, much less inclined to discuss their symptoms and often refuse even to acknowledge that anything is wrong.

Of the current array of psychotherapies, one widely used form traces its origins to the "talking cure" of Joseph Breuer and Anna O., discussed in Chapter 1. This treatment, which is based on the psychoanalytic approach, is called psychodynamic psychotherapy because it is concerned with the dynamic struggle of internal psychological forces. Patients are encouraged to discuss the meaning of their symptoms as reflections of unconscious mental processes that are expressed in symbolic forms, like those we use in our dreams. Symptoms, like dreams, are taken to be disguised enactments of internal wishes and conflicts. For example, the patient who feared he had hit someone with his car might be assumed to be struggling with intense aggressive impulses, the true object and origin of which would be discovered in the course of treatment. The central goal is to gain insight into the meaning of the symptoms and also into maladaptive interpersonal relationships, as reenacted with the therapist.

Whereas psychodynamic psychotherapy (along with its more elaborate form, psychoanalysis) has enjoyed wide popularity, it has not proven to be of much help in the management of the truly disabling anxiety disorders, such as panic disorder or OCD. John Nemiah, editor of the *American Journal of Psychiatry*, has made this point well with respect to OCD:

> It is one of the ironies of clinical psychiatry that, although the obsessive-compulsive disorder illuminates the psychoanalytic concept of psychodynamic conflict perhaps better than any other psychoneurosis, its symptoms generally remain impervious to psychoanalytic treatment. To the clinical observer, the patient's struggles with his unacceptable aggressive and scatological impulses, the intense anxiety they arouse in him, and the variety of defenses he employs to control them are all evidence of an intense internal psychic struggle. Unfortunately, such insight, even when it is shared by the patient, seems to have little or no effect on the course of symptoms, and until the advent of newer forms of treatment, patients suffering from obsessive-compulsive disorders were often doomed to a lifetime of painful and debilitating illness.

Other therapeutic approaches have been developed for patients with anxiety disorders that do not concern themselves with the symbolic meaning of symptoms but, instead, with techniques designed to eliminate them. Because the abnormal behavior is addressed directly, these approaches are called behavioral therapies. For example, phobic symptoms have been successfully attacked by means of a behavioral technique called systematic desensitization. The general approach is to have the patient gradually engage the feared object or commit the feared action, first mentally and then in progressively more real circumstances. Systematic desensitization is especially effective with simple phobias, such as fear of flying.

In many patients, a combination of psychotherapy and drug treatment has proved effective. Often, the drugs attenuate the anxiety sufficiently to make the patient receptive to the psychological treatment, which may then reduce or eliminate the need for medications.

Future Directions

In the past decade, our view of the anxiety disorders has changed dramatically. Traditionally, these conditions were considered to be primarily of psychological rather than biological origin. Of course, the role of "constitutional factors" was hard to dismiss; but the emphasis was on understanding psychological causes and improving psychological treatments.

Now, however, there is a growing amount of evidence arguing that genes play a role in causing anxiety disorders. Furthermore, drugs are being recognized as particularly effective forms of treatment. As a result of these developments, the most serious anxiety disorders—OCD and panic disorder—have now taken their places alongside mood disorders and schizophrenia as subjects for further biological investigation. Once again, the molecular approach would seem to have a great deal to offer.

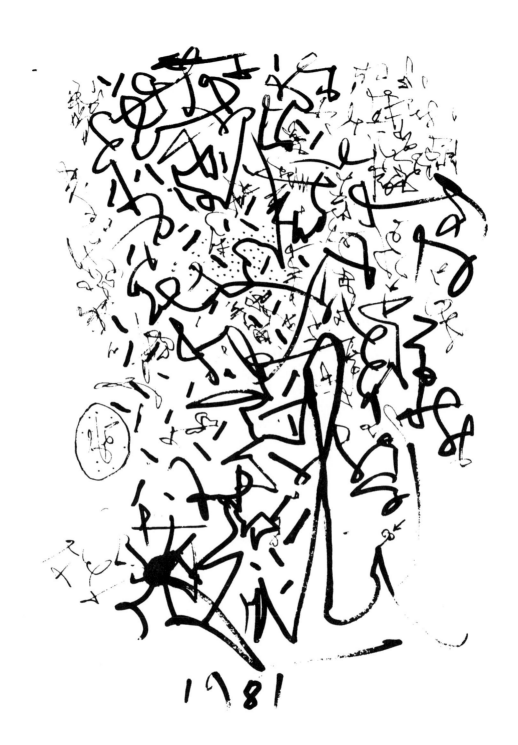

9

EPILOGUE

We began this book by considering Freud's ambition to contribute to a natural science of behavior by "represent[ing] psychical processes as quantitatively determinate states of specifiable material particles." We then saw him reluctantly give up this reductionist approach to psychiatric problems, choosing thereafter to address the psychological meaning of his patients' symptoms directly. In a letter written to his friend Wilhelm Fliess in 1895, Freud expressed intense disappointment at his failure satisfactorily to explain psychological phenomena in neuronal terms: ". . . After an excess of mental torment, I just apathetically tell myself that it does not hang together yet and perhaps never will. . . . The mechanical explanation is not coming off, and I am inclined to listen to the still, small voice which tells me that my explanation will not do."

OPPOSITE: Salvador Dali's portrayal of the complex structure of neurons and the interactions of their axonal and dendritic extensions, prepared for a celebration in memory of his countryman Santiago Ramón y Cajal.

In the century since Freud came to this conclusion, there has been a virtual explosion in our knowledge of biological factors that influence normal and abnormal behavior. We have learned a great deal about the detailed structure of the neurons that so fascinated Freud, and about their means of signaling each other. We have developed an impressive array of drugs that alleviate serious mental disturbances, as well as new (and less haphazard) approaches to finding still better ones. It will probably not be long before we are able to identify specific genes that give rise to certain forms of serious mental illness.

Over the course of this book we have looked at many of these advances in some detail. Now is the time to take stock of our present state of knowledge about neurons, genes, and drugs as it relates to mental illness; and, like Freud before us, place our bets on what are likely to be the most fruitful approaches in the foreseeable future.

Neurons

As Freud began to formulate ideas about mental mechanisms, he tried thinking of them in terms of neuronal interactions. For example, he made an attempt to conceptualize the process he called repression in the accompanying sketch of hypothetical neurons from *Project for a Scientific Psychology* (1895). But, as Freud properly concluded, he was not in a position to progress from this heuristic conception to explaining actual thoughts in

Freud's conceptualization of the psychological process of repression of a painful memory in terms of the flow of information in hypothetical neurons. In this diagram neuron *a*, which records "a hostile mnemic image," is under the control of neuron α, and *b* is "key-neuron to unpleasure," so that "with an inhibitory action from α the release of unpleasure will turn out very slight."

terms of real neuronal processes. Simply not enough was known about neurons to make the leap.

Since 1895 there has been an enormous growth of knowledge about neurons and the way they interact. Many of the molecular elements involved in neuronal signaling have been identified. We now know of dozens of neurotransmitters and the complex chain of postsynaptic events they control, from the opening and closing of ion channels, to activation of G proteins, to sending forth second messengers. We may even be on the verge of identifying alterations in the expression of specific neuronal genes, in response to repeated synaptic signaling, that lead to the storage of memories in the fabric of the brain. The outlines of the brain's innate wiring diagram are becoming clearer as knowledge accumulates about molecules on the surface of neurons that guide them in the selection of partners for synaptic connections.

We are also beginning to understand the rules that govern complicated neuronal circuits whose interactions produce such discernable mental processes as visual perception. This work is developing into a subspecialty, called integrative or systems neuroscience, that seeks to generate models of organized brain functions. More than molecular studies alone, systems neuroscience addresses issues that Freud would have been at home with. But it remains difficult to tackle such higher and complex mental functions as "repression." Integrative studies will ultimately be of enormous value; but for now, genes and drugs are easier to study, and work being done in those areas holds out greater hope for near-term practical advances in the understanding and management of mental illness.

Genes

At present, a search for genes that cause or predispose to mental illness seems particularly promising, thanks to the recent development of techniques for systematically searching through the human genome. We have already reviewed the general approach that should make it possible to ferret out the gene or genes that cause a well-defined mental illness such as bipolar disorder. We should then be able to study how the normal and abnormal alleles of these genes function in neurons, and how such functioning contributes to the expression of a mood disorder. Gene identification will also make it possible to reclassify mental illnesses in categories based on explicit causes rather than on clinical symptoms alone.

Despite the obvious value of genetic research, many people have expressed concern about its potentially undesirable social consequences. One danger is that a genetic point of view may be misused to justify social and racial inequities. But perverse social and political movements antedate, and are explicitly repudiated by, advances in genetics. The misuse of truth should not become the basis for inhibiting a search for disease genes by scientists who are fully cognizant of the limits of their approach and of the critical impact of environmental factors on all aspects of our lives.

Our growing ability directly to measure specific genes in individual people does, however, make possible new abuses. There is the danger, for example, that governments might be pressured to stamp out alleles of many genes, including those related to mood disorders or schizophrenia, by eliminating their citizens' reproductive choice. There is also the danger that people might be subjected to genetic screening to determine qualifications for a variety of opportunities, ranging from insurance, to jobs, to high political office. Fortunately, these ethical concerns are receiving great attention from the organizations committed to the detailed study of the human genome.

Drugs

While work on the genetics of mental illness is enormously promising, the most immediate payoffs will come from continued development of drugs. Psychopharmacology has already yielded many valuable products for the management of a wide range of behavioral disorders; and because a great deal is already known about the site of action of drugs at neuronal receptors and transporters, the discovery of new types of active compounds will be facilitated. Furthermore, technological advances are helping us to identify more variants of receptors with which drugs interact, setting the stage for the development of even more selective compounds.

Of course, there are problems here as well. For one thing, we remain ignorant about the long-term changes in the brain that accompany sustained drug intake. Such changes are responsible for certain therapeutic effects, such as the antidepressant action of imipramine, as well as for certain toxic side effects, such as the movement disorders caused by many antipsychotics. Further advances in psychopharmacology may well depend on understanding these long-term effects. We will need to analyze complex molecular regulatory mechanisms in the brain, not merely understand the simple interaction of a drug with an identified protein.

Because it has been so difficult to predict the overall effects of drugs on the brain, many drug discoveries, as we have repeatedly seen, have been accidental. It is not unlikely that we will benefit from more accidental discoveries in the future. There is also good reason to hope that identifying a gene responsible for a particular mental illness may point the way to new drugs that target the specific abnormality that the gene produces. The tripartite marriage of pharmacology with molecular biology and protein chemistry that has become stronger in the past few decades will make possible rapid exploitation of new leads, whatever their origin.

"Like Short Stories . . ."

Freud gave up his pursuit of a biological psychiatry not only because he felt the approach was premature. He also found it impossible to escape the fact that we do not really experience our lives in terms of "specifiable material particles." Our conscious impressions are, instead, of thinking and feeling. The forces that shape our actions are cultural, parental, and circumstantial. Human behavior lends itself better to metaphors drawn from these sources than to specific descriptions of the movement of signals through neuronal networks. Our lives, as Freud said, "read like short stories."

Although Freud never abandoned his conviction that neurons were ultimately important, he decided to analyze these stories in terms of a different set of elements—instincts, personality traits, defensive styles, learned skills. Furthermore, because of his scientific background, he assumed that the stories were lawful rather than random, and he searched for the rules that govern their narrative elements. Needless to say, this task has turned out to be no less challenging than unraveling the secrets of neuronal circuits or the molecular structure of neurons. Even today Freud would have to conclude that his system of psychological explanations also "does not hang together yet."

While recognizing the importance of uncovering rules that govern the behavior of the whole person, the main point of this book is that there is, at present, great practical value to examining factors that influence behavior at the molecular level. Of course, molecular science will never be up to the task of explaining the content of a person's short stories. But molecules are the ultimate stuff our short stories are made of; and, for now, the new knowledge being accumulated by a molecular approach offers the considerable promise of many more happy endings.

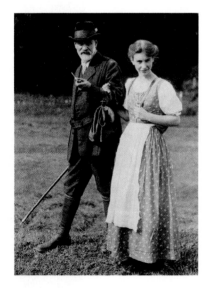

Sigmund Freud with his daughter Anna, also a psychoanalyst, in 1913.

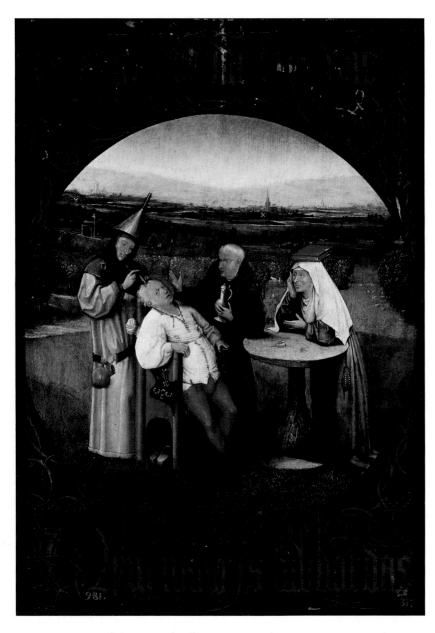

Extraction of the Stone of Folly, 1475–1480, by Hieronymus Bosch.

RECAPITULATION *(In Verse)*

I. Freud

"The problem is," young Sigmund said,
"To analyze these fish,
To take their spinal neurons out
And put them in a dish,
And see if my experiments
Disclose the things I wish."

("I justify this exercise
Because I'm now inclined
To think like a reductionist,
And trust that I will find
Within these simple neurons
Little secrets of the mind.")

But then he talked to Breuer
And he heard of Anna O.

And he learned to do hypnosis
From a Frenchman named Charcot.
And he thought, "With these new methods
I will *definitely* find
Not just tiny little secrets
But the *meaning* of the mind."

"Who cares if Dr. Ehrlich's drug
Has caused a great sensation,
Eradicating syphilis
To worldwide celebration.
For me a patient's stories
Are sufficient inspiration;
And *my* mighty 'magic bullet'
Is a dream interpretation!"

II. Drugs

The problem for the chemists
Was explicitly defined.
Just synthesize a lot of drugs
And hope that you will find
A patentable compound (that
Will benefit mankind).

So they made some novel structures
In some novel permutations,
And multiple derivatives
In strange configurations,
Which gave them many chemicals
That no one else had seen,
Including something special called
A phenothiazine.

Which, much to their amazement,
(And their company's great gain)
Was accidentally found to cause
Marked changes in the brain,
Deleting the delusions
Of the chronically insane.

Oh, what a stir these chemists caused
In finding this new potion.
Their seminal discovery
Set others into motion
(Perhaps there were some chemicals
That, in the proper doses,
Might prove to be superior
In clearing up psychosis).

And so they mixed more mixtures,
Manufactured variations,
And conjured up imipramine
By these improvisations;
Which didn't help psychosis
But gave other welcome news:
That a bottle of imipramine
Obliterates the blues!

Then other types of drugs were found
With other applications,

Like lithium's preventing both
Depressions and elations;
But great confusion followed from
This flood of information
(Since cures caused by these compounds
Came without an explanation).

Till they found a simple answer
(But an incomplete solution):
Most drugs must bind receptors,
Making simple substitution
For a natural transmitter
With such specificity
The receptor grants admittance
(As a lock admits a key).

And so, for schizophrenia,
(Whose key is dopamine),
You give a strong antagonist
(The phenothiazine)
That binds a D receptor, thereby
Getting in between
A site on the receptor
And the catecholamine.

It's different with depression—
There you bind amine transporters
That translocate transmitters
(Which makes their actions shorter);
And by yet another tactic
You may switch from fright to fight
By increasing GABA's binding
To a GABA binding site.

So praise the clever chemists
For the drugs they have confected
(Since changing minds with chemicals
Was really unexpected).
Now, with their new technology
That's sure to expedite
Additional discoveries—
All minds may soon work right.

Recapitulation (in Verse)

III. Genes

The problem solved by Mendel was
Why yellow peas, or green,
Could be either smooth or wrinkled,
Which he understood to mean:
That the color and the texture
Each reflects a different gene.

But far beyond the reach of even
Mendel's intuition,
There lurked the well-kept secrets of
Genetic composition:
The nature of the stuff used in
Genetic fabrication;
And the nature of the rules that rule
Genetic replication.

But behold nucleic acids, and
The secret is exposed,
And the rules of replication can be
Finally proposed,
And the meaning of base pairing
Can be rapidly revealed,
Since the bases tell the story
(That was cunningly concealed).

For the code of replication is
Determined by the places
That are copied in transcription
(By touching all four bases),
In that A and T, or G and C
Perform a clever trick,
By being complementary
(As Watson is to Crick).

And three of them, in order,
Lead to literal translation
In amino acid language
That transmits this declamation
To a hundred thousand proteins

That complete the transmutation
From the sequence of the bases
Into protein conformation.

But beware a single error
In the linear array
Of As and Ts, or Gs and Cs,
Whose orderly display
Is absolutely needed
Lest there be a misquotation
That causes odd behavior
From molecular mutation.

For instance, in a fruit fly
If the error is in *per*
It dysregulates some rhythms
So the wings won't rightly whir;
And a mutant human enzyme
Can bring total devastation
To the elegant progression
Of our cerebral formation.

So, given these examples,
The task becomes to seek
(By proper application
Of molecular technique)
The genes that cause such problems
As obsessional neurosis,
Severe agoraphobia,
Delusional psychosis.

For once a gene's discovered
And is captured in a clone,
The protein that it codes for is
Immediately known,
Unleashing all the power of
Molecular biology
To exorcise the demons of
Behavioral pathology.

IV. Stories

The problem that remains is that,
Despite these revelations,
A science based on molecules
Has latent limitations
That limit its capacity
To serve as a notation
For thoughts that we experience
In our imagination.

For lives are lived as stories
(Though their intrapsychic actors
May play from scripts whose scripting comes
From polygenic factors);
And lives are understandable
In terms of mental rules
(Though they respond, like puppets,
To key protein molecules).

But should a plot develop
That is different than expected,
And should a role have features
That the player wants corrected,

That role may prove refractory
To thespian intention,
While chemicals may constitute
The proper intervention.

So even though our stories are
Intangible, ethereal,
Our mental composition is
Essentially material;
And though we don't experience
This transubstantiation,
To know ourselves requires
Its detailed elucidation.

And not just to design some
More effective medications,
But also to define a view
With wider implications,
Since understanding molecules
That drive us to insanity
Provides a giant window on
The nature of humanity.

FURTHER READINGS

Alberts, Bruce, Dennis Bray, Julian Lewis, Martin Raff, Keith Roberts, and James D. Watson. *Molecular Biology of the Cell*. 2d edition. New York: Garland Publishing, 1989.

Cooper, Jack R., Floyd E. Bloom, and Robert H. Roth. *The Biochemical Basis of Neuropharmacology*. 6th edition. New York: Oxford University Press, 1991.

Gelehrter, Thomas D., and Francis S. Collins. *Principles of Medical Genetics*. Baltimore: Williams and Wilkins, 1990.

Goodwin, Frederick K., and Kay Redfield Jamison. *Manic-Depressive Illness*. New York: Oxford University Press, 1990.

Gottesman, Irving I. *Schizophrenia Genesis*. New York: W. H. Freeman and Company, 1991.

Griffiths, Anthony J. F., Jeffrey H. Miller, David T. Suzuki, Richard C. Lewontin, and William M. Gelbart. *An Introduction to Genetic Analysis*. 5th edition. New York: W. H. Freeman and Company, 1993.

Hall, Zach W. *An Introduction to Molecular Neurobiology*. Sunderland, Mass.: Sinauer Associates, 1992.

Kandel, Eric, James H. Schwartz, and Thomas Jessell. *Principles of Neural Science*. 3d edition. New York: Elsevier Science Publishing, 1991.

Plomin, Robert, J. C. DeFries, and G. E. McClearn. *Behavioral Genetics*. 2d edition. New York: W. H. Freeman and Company, 1990.

Rapoport, Judith L. *The Boy Who Couldn't Stop Washing*. New York: New American Library, 1990.

Sulloway, Frank J. *Freud, Biologist of the Mind*. New York: Basic Books, 1979.

Watson, James D., Michael Gilman, Jan Witkowski, and Mark Zoller. *Recombinant DNA*. 2d edition. New York: Scientific American Books, 1992.

REFERENCES AND SOURCES OF ILLUSTRATIONS

Original drawings by Gabor Kiss and Tomo Narashima; charts and graphs by FineLine Illustrations.

Cover image: Collection de l'art brut, Lausanne.

Page ii: Prado, Madrid. Scala/Art Resource.

Chapter 1   *Page x:* Edimedia.   *Page 4:* Drawing from Sigmund Freud, "Über Spinalganglien und Rückenmark des Petromyzon," *Sitzungsberichte der kaiserlichen Akademie der Wissenschaften* (Wien). Mathematisch Naturwissenschaftliche Classe, 78, III. Abteilung:81–167, 1878. Quotation from *The Standard Edition of the Complete Psychological Works of Sigmund Freud* (London: Hogarth Press) 1:295.   *Page 5:* André Brouillet, *A Lesson by Dr. Jean-Martin Charcot at the Salpêtrière Hospital.* Erich Lessing/Art Resource.   *Page 6:* Richard Bergh, *Hypnotic Séance,* 1887. Nationalmuseum, Stockholm.   *Page 7:* Institut für Geschichte der Medizin der Universität Wien.   *Page 8:* Stadtarchiv, Frankfurt am Main.   *Page 9:* Freud, *Standard Edition* 2:160.   *Page 11:* Ibid. 18:60.   *Page 12:* STD Division, Centers for Disease Control.   *Page 13:* (*Top*) Bettmann Archive; (*bottom*) Warner Brothers, © 1940 Turner Entertainment Co.   *Page 16:* Imperial War Museum/E. T. Archive.   *Page 17:* National Library of Medicine.

Chapter 2   *Page 20:* Peter Lichter et al., *Science* 247(1990): 64–69; © 1990 by AAAS.   *Page 22:* Charles Darwin, *The Descent of Man and Selection in Relation to Sex* (London: John Murray, 1871), 414.   *Page 34:* (*Left*) Nathaniel Currier. New-York Historical Society; (*right*) Eastman Johnson, 1846. National Portrait Gallery, Washington, D.C./Art Resource.   *Page 35:* (*Left*) Mathew Brady, 1860. National Portrait Gallery, Washington, D.C./Art Resource; (*right*) Massachusetts Historical Society.   *Pages 36, 37:* From C. P. Kyriacou and J. C. Hall, *Proceedings of the National Academy of Sciences* 77 (1980): 6729–33.   *Page 39:* Sir Edwin Landseer, *Dignity and Impudence,* 1839. Tate Gallery, London/Art Resource.   *Page 41:* Adapted from J. C. DeFries, M. C. Gervais, and E. A. Thomas, *Behavior Genetics* 8(1978): 3–13.   *Page 42:* Drawing by Chas. Addams; © 1981 The New Yorker Magazine, Inc.

Chapter 3   *Page 44:* Cold Spring Harbor Laboratory Archives.   *Page 61:* Adapted from David T. Suzuki et al., *An Introduction to Genetic Analysis,* 4th edition (New York: W. H. Freeman, 1989), 433.

Chapter 4   *Page 64:* Nancy Kedersha, ImmunoGen, Inc., Cambridge, Mass. The red stain is linked to an antibody that binds to a protein that is expressed only in neurons. The blue stain binds to DNA in all cell nuclei and indicates the presence in the tissue culture dish of supporting cells that help prepare a surface on which the neurons grow.   *Page 69:* Mary Ann Martone, David Hessler, and Mark Ellisman/San Diego Microscopy and Imaging Resource, University of California, San Diego.   *Page 70:* Electron micrograph from C. Raine, in G. J. Siegel et al., *Basic Neurochemistry,* 3d edition (Boston: Little, Brown, 1981), 32.   *Page 73:* Adapted from W. J. Freeman, *Scientific American* 264 (February 1991): 78–85.   *Page 86:* Julie Newdoll, Computer Graphics Laboratory, UCSF. © Regents, University of California.

Chapter 5   *Page 90:* Michelangelo Merisi da Caravaggio, *Bacchus,* 1589. Uffizi, Florence/E. T. Archive.   *Page 94:* Reese T. Jones in C. N. Chiang and R. L. Hawks, *Research Findings on Smoking of Abused Substances* (NIDA Research Monograph 99) (Washington, D.C.: U.S. Government Printing Office, 1990), 30–41.   *Page 96:* J. Stephenson and J. M. Churchill, *Medical Botany* (London, 1836), vol. 3, plate 136. New York Botanical Garden Library.   *Page 97:* J. Stephenson and J. M. Churchill, *Medical Botany* (London, 1834), vol. 1, plate 1. New York Botanical Garden Library.   *Page 98:* Julie Newdoll, Computer Graphics Laboratory, UCSF. © Regents, University of California.   *Page 102:* Pierre Deniker in F. J. Ayd and B. Blackwell, eds., *Discoveries in Biological Psychiatry* (Philadelphia: J. B. Lippincott, 1970), 157.   *Page 104:* Photograph courtesy of Solomon Snyder; quotation from Roland Kuhn in *Discoveries in Biological Psychiatry,* 211.   *Page 114:* Sabina Berretta and Ann Graybiel, *Journal of Neurophysiology* 68 (1992): 767–77.

Chapter 6   *Page 116:* Vincent van Gogh, *Self-portrait with gray felt hat,* 1887. Rijksmuseum, Amsterdam.   *Page 119:* Herman Melville, *Billy Budd and Other Stories* (New York: Viking Penguin, 1986), 353.   *Page 120:* Sylvia Plath, *The Bell Jar* (New York: Harper & Row, 1971) 142. R. R. Fieve, *Moodswing* (New York: William Morrow, 1975), 148.   *Pages 121–23 Diagnostic and Statistical Manual of Mental Disorders,* 3d edition, revised (Washington, D.C.: American Psychiatric Association, 1987), xxii.   *Page 122:* (*Top*) K. Squillace, R. M. Post,

210

R. Savard, and M. Erwin-Gorman in R. M. Post and J. C. Ballenger, eds., *Neurobiology of Mood Disorders* (Baltimore: Williams and Wilkins, 1984), 44; (*bottom*) adapted from F. K. Goodwin and K. R. Jamison, *Manic-Depressive Illness* (New York, Oxford University Press, 1990), 81. *Page 124: DSM-III-R,* 217. *Page 125:* Ibid., 222. *Page 126:* (*Left*) Attrib. J. Closterman; (*right*) Walter Richard Sickert, 1927. Both National Portrait Gallery, London. Quotation from Anthony Storr, *Churchill's Black Dog, Kafka's Mice, and Other Phenomena of the Human Mind* (New York: Grove Press, 1988), 15. *Page 127:* Vincent van Gogh, 1889. Stedelijk Museum, Amsterdam. *Page 128:* Estimates of the incidence of bipolar disorder and major depression were derived by combining data from several studies summarized in Goodwin and Jamison, *Manic-Depressive Illness,* 379. *Page 130:* Jerry Irwin. *Page 131:* Derived from Janice A. Egeland and Abram A. Hostetter, *American Journal of Psychiatry* 140 (1983): 56–61. *Page 132:* Julie Newdoll, Computer Graphics Laboratory, UCSF. © Regents, University of California. *Page 133:* (*Top*) © 1990, Newsweek, Inc.; (*bottom*) Julie Newdoll, Computer Graphics Laboratory, UCSF. © Regents, University of California. *Pages 137–38:* John F. J. Cade in *Discoveries in Biological Psychiatry,* 223. *Page 139:* Adapted from P.C. Baastrup and M. Schou, *Archives of General Psychiatry* 16 (1967): 162–72.

Chapter 7 *Page 142:* Prinzhorn Collection, Heidelberg. *Pages 146, 147:* National Library of Medicine. *Pages 148–49: DSM-III-R,* 193–94. *Page 150:* Adapted from I. I. Gottesman, *Schizophrenia Genesis* (New York: W. H. Freeman, 1991) 96. *Page 151:* Edna Morloc. *Page 152:* Adapted from Suzuki, *Genetic Analysis,* 5th edition, 103. Page 153: National Institute of Mental Health; from a study by R. L. Suddath, G. W. Christison, E. F. Torrey, M. F. Casanova, and D. R. Weinberger, *New England Journal of Medicine* 322 (1990):789–94. *Pages 158, 160:* Julie Newdoll, Computer Graphics Laboratory, UCSF. © Regents, University of California. *Page 162:* T. Van-Putten, S. R. Marder, W. C. Wirshing, M. Aravakagiri, and N. Chabert, *Schizophrenia Bulletin* 17 (1991): 197–216. *Page 164:* L. Farde, A.-L. Nordström, F.-A. Wiesel, S. Pauli, C. Halldin, and G. Sedvall, *Archives of General Psychiatry,* 49 (July 1992) 541. *Page 165:* After Philip

Seeman, *Journal of NIH Research* 3 (1991): 58. The amino acid sequence and the predicted transmembrane segments are from H. H. M. Van Tol et al., *Nature* 350 (1991): 610–614. *Page 167:* Sherman Bailey Weisburd, courtesy of Dan E. Weisburd.

Chapter 8 *Page 172:* Prado, Madrid. Scala/Art Resource. *Page 174:* N. Tinbergen, *The Herring Gull's World* (New York: Basic Books, 1960), 215. *Page 175: Cat Terrified at a Dog.* From life, by Mr. Wood. In Charles Darwin, *The Expression of the Emotions in Man and Animals* (London: John Murray, 1872). American Museum of Natural History, New York. *Pages 176–77: DSM-III-R,* 9. *Page 178:* Data for graph from L. N. Robins and D. A. Regier, eds., *Psychiatric Disorders in America: The Epidemiologic Catchment Area Study* (New York: Free Press, York, 1991). *Pages 180–81:* Nancy C. Andreasen, *The Broken Brain* (New York: Harper & Row, 1984), 65–66. *Page 182:* Sigmund Freud, *A General Introduction to Psychoanalysis,* Seventeenth Lecture (New York: Washington Square Press, 1960), 270. *Pages 182–83:* James Boswell, *The Life of Dr. Johnson,* (London: J. M. Dent & Sons, 1933), 301–302. *Page 183:* (*Left*) Sir Joshua Reynolds, c. 1756. National Portrait Gallery, London; (*right*) Smithsonian Institution/National Air and Space Museum. *Pages 184–85:* Judith L. Rapoport, *The Boy Who Couldn't Stop Washing* (New York: NAL/Dutton, 1990), 21–24. *Page 187:* Thomas Uhde, National Institutes of Health. *Page 189:* (*Left*) Dirck Halstead/Black Star; (*right*) Raymond Depardon/MAGNUM. *Page 191:* Julie Newdoll, Computer Graphics Laboratory, UCSF. © Regents, University of California. *Page 196:* J. C. Nemiah in T. R. Insel, ed., *New Findings in Obsessive Compulsive Disorder* (Washington, D.C.: American Psychiatric Press, 1984), ix.

Chapter 9 *Page 198:* Instituto de Investigaciones Citologicas, Valencia. *Page 199:* Sigmund Freud, *The Origins of Psycho-Analysis: Letters to Wilhelm Fliess, Drafts and Notes, 1887–1902* (New York: Basic Books, 1954), 126. *Page 200:* Drawing from Freud, *Standard Edition* 1: 324. *Page 203:* Sigmund Freud Archives/Mary Evans Picture Library, Courtesy of W. E. Freud. **Recapitulation (in Verse)** Page 204: Prado, Madrid. Scala/Art Resource.

INDEX

Acetylcholine, 75, 76, 81–82, 83, 98–99
Action potential, 77
Adenine, 46
Adenylate cyclase, 86
Agonists, 95–96
  inverse, 191
  partial, 99
Agoraphobia, 178, 179–181
Akathisia, 161
Akinesia, 161
Alcohol, GABA receptors and, 193–194
Allele, 24–25
Allosteric protein, 53
Alprazolam (Xanax), 190
Amanita muscaria, 96
Amino acids
  neurotransmitter, 80–81
  in protein synthesis, 50–52, 60
Amphetamine, 155–157
Anions, in electrical signaling, 75
Antagonists, 95–97
Antianxiety agents, 188–194
Anticodon, 51
Antidepressants
  development of, 104–105, 206
  mechanism of action of, 133–136
  for obsessive-compulsive disorder, 194–195
Antipsychotic drugs, 100–105, 106, 159–166, 206
  dopamine receptors and, 159–166
  movement abnormalities and, 160–163, 164
Anxiety
  generalized, 179
  performance, 188–189
  signal, 175
Anxiety disorders, 173–197
  behavioral therapy for, 196–197
  characteristics of, 177–183
  drug therapy for, 188–195
  genetic factors in, 187
  neurosis and, 175–177
  prevalence of, 177–178
  psychotherapy for, 195–196
Anxiolytics, 188–194

Arsphenamine (Salvarsan), 15
Atropa belladonna, 97
Atropine, 97–99
Autosomal dominant inheritance, 22, 28
Autosomal recessive inheritance, 29, 31–32
Autosomes, 24
Avoidance behavior, physiology of, 173–175
Axons, 68, 69, 72

Baldness, male-pattern, 34–35
Barbiturates, GABA receptors and, 193–194
Base pairing, 46–48, 207
  in genetic diagnosis, 61–63
Base sequences, variations in, 60
Behavior, open-field, 40
Behavioral inheritance, 21–43
  in dogs, 40
  in mice, 40
  multiple-gene, 38–42
  single-gene, 35–38
  twin studies of, 41–42
Behavioral therapy, for anxiety disorders, 196–197
Belladonna, 97
Benzodiazepines, for anxiety, 190–194
Beta-blockers, for anxiety, 188–189
Biological psychiatry
  definition of, 1
  Freud's abandonment of, 3–9, 199–201, 203
  limitations of, 203, 208
  social and ethical aspects of, 202
  trends in, 2–3
Bipolar disorder, 122, 123–131. *See also* Depression; Mania
  diagnostic criteria for, 124
  electroconvulsive therapy for, 139–140
  genetic factors in, 128–129
  lithium for, 137–139, 206
  prevalence of, 123
  treatment trends in, 140–141

Bleuler, Eugen, 146, 147
Brain abnormalities, in schizophrenia, 153–154
Brain changes, drug-induced, 112–114
Brain disease, psychiatric symptoms in, 12–17
Breuer, Josef, 7–9, 205
Brücke, Ernst, 3–4

Calcium, in cell signaling, 74–79
Canine acral lick, 195
Carbamazepine, 139
Catatonic schizophrenia, 146
Catecholamines, anxiety and, 188–190
cDNA library, 110–112, 113
Cell-to-cell signaling, 69–70, 74
Channel-linked receptors, 84
Charcot, Jean-Martin, 5, 6
Chlordiazepoxide (Librium), 190
Chloride, in cell signaling, 74–79
Chlorpromazine
  for mania, 138
  receptor binding of, 107–109
  for schizophrenia, 101–103, 105, 106, 160
Cholecystokinin, 81
Cholinergic receptors, 99
Chromosomes, 20, 24–28
  crossovers of, 25–28, 60
  definition of, 23
  homologous, 24
  nonhomologous, 24
  sex, 24
Churchill, John, 126, 127
Churchill, Randolph, 12, 126–127
Churchill, Winston, 126–127
Clomipramine, 194–195
Cloning, of receptors, 109–112, 113
Clozapine (Clozaril), 159, 161–166
Cocaine, 114, 155–156
Codons, 50–51, 60
Cognitive therapy, 140–141
Complementary DNA (cDNA), 110, 111, 113

Compulsions. *See* Obsessive-compulsive disorder
Concentration gradient, 75
Conversion disorder, 5–11
Corticotropin-releasing factor, 81
Cortisol, 136
Crack. *See* Cocaine
Crick, Francis, 44, 46–47, 207
Crossing over, 25–28, 60
Curare, 99
Cyclic AMP, 85, 86
Cyclothymia, 123
Cytoplasm, 66
Cytosine, 46
Cytoskeleton, 66

Darwin, Charles, 21–22
Delusions, in schizophrenia, 144, 148
Dementia paralytica, 12–15
Dementia praecox, 145
Dendrites, 68, 69, 72
Dense core vesicles, 82
Deoxyribonucleic acid. *See* DNA
Dependence, drug, 194
Depolarization, 75–78
Depression, 122, 123–131. *See also* Bipolar disorder; Mood disorders
  cortisol and, 136
  diagnostic criteria for, 124
  drug therapy for, 103–106, 132–135, 206
  electroconvulsive therapy for, 139–140
  in pellagra, 16–17
Desensitization, 114
Desipramine, 134
Diacylglycerol, 87, 138–139
Diagnostic and Statistical Manual of Mental Disorders (DSM-III-R), 121–123, 176–177
Diazepam (Valium), 190, 191
Diazepam binding inhibitor, 193
Dimethyltryptamine (DMT), 155
Direct binding assays, 107–109
Disorganized schizophrenia, 146

Other Books in the Scientific American Library Series

POWERS OF TEN
by Philip and Phylis Morrison and the Office of
Charles and Ray Eames

HUMAN DIVERSITY
by Richard Lewontin

THE DISCOVERY OF SUBATOMIC
PARTICLES
by Steven Weinberg

FOSSILS AND THE HISTORY OF LIFE
by George Gaylord Simpson

ON SIZE AND LIFE
by Thomas A. McMahon and John Tyler Bonner

FIRE
by John W. Lyons

SUN AND EARTH
by Herbert Friedman

ISLANDS
by H. William Menard

DRUGS AND THE BRAIN
by Solomon H. Synder

THE TIMING OF BIOLOGICAL CLOCKS
by Arthur T. Winfree

EXTINCTION
by Steven M. Stanley

EYE, BRAIN, AND VISION
by David H. Hubel

THE SCIENCE OF STRUCTURES AND
MATERIALS
by J. E. Gordon

THE HONEY BEE
by James L. Gould and Carol Grant Gould

ANIMAL NAVIGATION
by Talbot H. Waterman

SLEEP
by J. Allan Hobson

FROM QUARKS TO THE COSMOS
by Leon M. Lederman and David N. Schramm

SEXUAL SELECTION
by James L. Gould and Carol Grant Gould

THE NEW ARCHAEOLOGY AND THE
ANCIENT MAYA
by Jeremy A. Sabloff

A JOURNEY INTO GRAVITY AND
SPACETIME
by John Archibald Wheeler

SIGNALS
by John R. Pierce and A. Michael Noll

BEYOND THE THIRD DIMENSION
by Thomas F. Banchoff

DISCOVERING ENZYMES
by David Dressler and Huntington Potter

THE SCIENCE OF WORDS
by George A. Miller

ATOMS, ELECTRONS, AND CHANGE
by P. W. Atkins

VIRUSES
by Arnold J. Levine

DIVERSITY AND THE TROPICAL RAIN
FOREST
by John Terborgh

STARS
by James B. Kaler

EXPLORING BIOMECHANICS
by R. McNeill Alexander

CHEMICAL COMMUNICATION
by William C. Agosta

GENES AND THE BIOLOGY OF CANCER
by Harold Varmus and Robert A. Weinberg

SUPERCOMPUTING
AND THE TRANSFORMATION OF SCIENCE
by William J. Kaufmann III and Larry L. Smarr